Epidural Analgesia in
Acute Pain Management

Epidural Analgesia in Acute Pain Management

Edited by

CAROLYN MIDDLETON

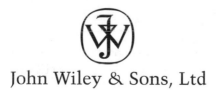

John Wiley & Sons, Ltd

Other Wiley Editorial Offices

John Wiley & Sons Inc., 111 River Street, Hoboken, NJ 07030, USA

Jossey-Bass, 989 Market Street, San Francisco, CA 94103-1741, USA

Wiley-VCH Verlag GmbH, Boschstr. 12, D-69469 Weinheim, Germany

John Wiley & Sons Australia Ltd, 42 McDougall Street, Milton, Queensland 4064, Australia

John Wiley & Sons (Asia) Pte Ltd, 2 Clementi Loop #02-01, Jin Xing Distripark, Singapore 129809

John Wiley & Sons Canada Ltd, 22 Worcester Road, Etobicoke, Ontario, Canada M9W 1L1

Wiley also publishes its books in a variety of electronic formats. Some content that appears in print may not be available in electronic books.

Epidural analgesia in acute pain management / editor,
   Carolyn Middleton.
      p. ; cm.
   Includes bibliographical references and index.
   ISBN-13: 978-0-470-01964-1 (pbk. : alk. paper)
   ISBN-10: 0-470-01964-6 (pbk. : alk. paper)
   1. Peridural anesthesia. 2. Analgesia. 3. Pain—Chemotherapy.
   I. Middleton, Carolyn.
      [DNLM: 1. Analgesia, Epidural—methods—Practice Guideline.
   2. Pain—prevention & control—Practice Guideline. WO 305 E64 2006]
   RD85.P4E65 2006
  617.9'64—dc22
A catalogue record for this book is available from the British Library

ISBN-13   978-0-470-01964-1
ISBN-10   0-470-01964-6

Typeset by SNP Best-set Typesetter Ltd., Hong Kong
Printed and bound in Great Britain by TJ International Ltd, Padstow, Cornwall

This book is printed on acid-free paper responsibly manufactured from sustainable forestry in which at least two trees are planted for each one used for paper production.

I dedicate this book to my family and friends

Contents

Contents

List of Figures

List of Tables

Contributors

Dee Comerford Clinical Nurse Specialist in Pain Management, Singleton Hospital, Swansea, South Wales

Lynda Jenkins Clinical Nurse Specialist in Pain Management, Morriston Hospital, Swansea, South Wales

Carolyn Middleton Clinical Nurse Specialist in Pain Management, Nevill Hall Hospital, Abergavenny, South Wales

Rachel Swinglehurst Clinical Nurse Specialist in Pain Management, Withybush Hospital, Pembrokeshire, South Wales

Foreword

Despite increasing popularity and significant scientific advances in relation to epidural analgesia, there appears to be a notable lack of published literature guiding this very specialised area of acute pain management practice. The aim of this book is to address this deficit by providing a clear practical but evidence-based pathway that describes in detail all aspects of epidural analgesia delivery in an acute secondary care setting. The text also addressed many Clinical Governance issues including risk management, evidence based practice, education, audit and research.

There is no doubt that if a modern safe and effective epidural service is to exist and flourish collaborative working between multiple disciplines is essential. It is therefore intended that this book should act as a useful resource for a variety of healthcare professionals including nurses, midwives, doctors, physiotherapists and pharmacists. The information presented will provide a comprehensive practical and theoretical guide for new staff members, a reference resource for experienced practitioners, and also a useful framework and template for epidural service development and delivery.

Carolyn Middleton MSc., BSc(Hons), RGN, Supplementary Prescriber.

Preface

The epidural space was first described in 1901 by Corning, and in 1921 Fidel used epidural anaesthesia in human beings. The first epidural was performed in the United Kingdom in the 1940s and since then numerous improvements in both equipment and drugs have taken place. Over the past two decades epidurals have become increasingly popular and versatile, with applications in adult surgery, trauma, obstetrics and paediatric practice. Epidural analgesia has been described as the gold standard of pain control, and, as relief of pain should be a fundamental objective of any health service, an epidural ward based provision is an essential addition to the analgesic armamentarium of every hospital.

Establishments such as the National Institute for Health and Clinical Excellence (NICE) provide evidence based guidance for the provision of care that is patient centred, cost effective and will attempt to reduce existing variations in practice. Currently NICE has not issued any such guidance for epidural practice, therefore the best practice guidelines presented within this book are designed to offer direction primarily to registered nurses, midwives and student nurses (but also to other members of the multidisciplinary healthcare team) in order to encourage a consistent and cohesive approach to epidural care.

The best practice guidelines were based on a document produced by the concerted inspiration and hard work of members of the South Wales Pain Nurses' Forum in collaboration with the Welsh Acute Pain Interest Group (my grateful thanks to all members of these two groups). A consensus development conference approach was used to collate and review epidural analgesia policies, protocols and practices from 11 hospitals in South Wales to identify commonalities and themes of clinical practice. Where literature was available it was critically appraised and in the absence of research evidence expert consensus of the group was reached. Thus best practice was agreed upon and the guideline document produced.

The purpose of this book of best practice guidelines for epidural analgesia in acute pain management is to promote the benefits of epidural analgesia while helping to minimise the risks. It is hoped that the information provided will be used as a basis for promoting effective interdisciplinary team working, to serve as a measure for quality in postoperative pain management and in doing so will help develop and improve patient care. It is also anticipated that the guidelines will stimulate learning among nursing teams and highlight ideas and priorities for nursing research.

The book can be used as a quick reference guide for clinical practice or as a framework for developing individual local epidural practice guidelines. The information provided is not intended to guide practice in palliative care or in the specialist management of persistent non-malignant pain.

Acknowledgements

My grateful thanks to all of those people who have helped to make this publication possible. Special thanks go to the three other contributors, Lynda Jenkins, Rachel Swinglehurst and Dee Comerford. Also on Dee's behalf I would like to thank Christine Court who helped with the literature search and preparation of Chapter 10.

Thanks to the individuals and bodies that have granted permission to reproduce previously published material. Also thanks to Gareth Middleton and B-Braun for many of the images provided.

I would like to particularly thank past and current members of the South Wales Pain Nurses' Forum (in collaboration with the Welsh Acute Pain Interest Group) for allowing me to take their original best practice framework and develop the concept into this book.

Finally thanks to both Whurr and Wiley publishers for their assistance.

1

Responsibilities of the Multidisciplinary Acute Pain Team

CAROLYN MIDDLETON

Clinical Nurse Specialist in Pain Management, Nevill Hall Hospital, Abergavenny, South Wales

Epidural analgesia is highly effective for controlling acute postoperative and trauma pain. The combination of excellent pain relief associated with minimal side effects provides high patient satisfaction when compared with other methods of analgesia. Epidurals can, however, cause serious, potentially life threatening complications and the safe, effective management of this type of intervention requires a coordinated multidisciplinary team approach (Royal College of Anaesthetists (RCA) and Association of Anaesthetists of Great Britain and Ireland (AAGBI), 2004).

Each member of the pain team must act in accordance with their own professional code and they must also follow local and national guidelines. The aim of this chapter is to outline individual specific responsibilities in relation to epidural analgesia.

Epidural Analgesia in Acute Pain Management. Edited by Carolyn Middleton.
© 2006 by John Wiley & Sons, Ltd. ISBN 0-470-01964-6

RESPONSIBILITIES OF THE ANAESTHETIST

RESPONSIBILITIES FOR THE ACUTE PAIN SERVICE

Following the publication of the joint report of the Royal Colleges of Surgeons and Anaesthetists (1990) many trusts have developed acute pain services in a bid to improve pain management for patients. This can be achieved through the implementation of ward based technical delivery systems such as epidural infusions (Bibby, 2001).

The development of an epidural service is predominantly anaesthesia led with the majority of research evidence on this subject emanating from anaesthetists. There should be a named consultant anaesthetist with a specific interest in pain management responsible for the supervision of the acute pain service within each hospital. He or she should have dedicated sessions allocated in order to carry out responsibilities which will include the provision of technical expert support and to review and synthesise current evidence into clinical practice. It is also necessary for the consultant to work closely with the clinical nurse specialist(s) (CNS) to develop and introduce clear protocols and guidelines to support an epidural ward based service.

ASSESSMENT OF PATIENT SUITABILITY FOR EPIDURAL ANALGESIA

The decision to provide epidural analgesia postoperatively is made by an anaesthetist with the patient's consent (see Chapter 2 for further information). The anaesthetist is uniquely qualified to assess the patient for regional analgesia and, while other professional groups may also be involved, it is the anaesthetist who provides the framework for practice.

Appropriate preoperative management of the patient is as important as postoperative monitoring. A detailed history and physical assessment is vital as preoperative preparation is one of the keys to success with regional anaesthesia and analgesia. The objectives of the anaesthetists, in relation to epidural patient selection, according to the Association of Anaesthetists of Great Britain and Ireland guidelines on preoperative assessment (2001), are to identify potential difficulties and existing medical conditions, and to improve safety by assessing and quantifying risk and by allowing planning of perioperative care.

It is also necessary for the anaesthetists to provide the patients with a careful explanation about the procedure (Chapter 3) which will aid the patient's co-operation making technical performance of epidural catheter insertion easier. The anaesthetists must provide the patient with an opportunity for explanation and discussion in order to allay fears and anxieties. Explanation is important as the Association of Anaesthetists of Great Britain and Ireland (2001) suggests that for a patient to wake up with an epidural in place that he or she has little or any understanding of comes as a surprise that may alarm the patient.

The anaesthetist's preoperative visit to the patient not only gives the opportunity for the assessment to take place; it also creates an environment of trust and confidence and allows a relationship between the patient and the anaesthetist to develop prior to their meeting in theatre.

INTRODUCTION AND MAINTENANCE OF THE EPIDURAL INFUSION

The anaesthetist has ultimate responsibility for introduction of the catheter into the epidural space under strict aseptic conditions (Chapter 3). He or she also has responsibility for prescribing an appropriate dosing regimen for both the initiation and continuation of the epidural infusion (Chapter 4). Alongside this prescription there should be balanced analgesia, a suitable antiemetic agent and the opioid antagonist naloxone prescribed on the patient's medication chart.

The anaesthetists should be involved in the decision making process regarding the appropriateness of discharging a patient with an epidural infusion in place from recovery back to a designated ward area. Often day-to-day review and management of the patient receiving an epidural infusion, after they have left recovery, is passed to the CNS (RCA and AAGBI, 2004).

SUPERVISION OF JUNIOR ANAESTHETIC STAFF

Ultimate responsibility for an epidural infusion must remain with the individual anaesthetist who instituted it, except in the case of trainees where the supervising consultant is accountable.

Doctors in training must possess defined competencies before performing epidural catheter insertions and establishing infusions without the direct supervision of a consultant or senior colleague (RCA and AAGBI, 2004). (Additional competencies are required when dealing with paediatric cases.) All required competencies are defined in the training manuals available from the RCA website (www.rcoa.ac.uk).

24 HOUR CONTINUING RESPONSIBILITY

In every hospital where an epidural service exists there should be 24 hour access to an anaesthetist for advice regarding the management of continuous epidural analgesia and its potentially serious associated side effects.

RECORD KEEPING

Anaesthetists are required to keep clear, accurate, legible and contemporaneous patients' records that report relevant clinical findings, decisions made, information given to patients and drugs prescribed (RCA and AAGBI, 2002). Accurate documentation enables the patient to receive effective continuing care because any member of the multidisciplinary team is able to assume care of the patient at any time with accurate up-to-date information available.

RESPONSIBILITIES OF THE SPECIALIST NURSE IN ACUTE PAIN MANAGEMENT

Following the joint report of the Royal College of Anaesthetists and the Royal College of Surgeons (1990), which highlighted the need for improving standards of postoperative pain management, a proliferation of 'acute pain teams' has arisen. This multidisciplinary pain management team, as part of its role, should oversee the delivery of epidural infusions throughout the hospital.

The team should include a clinical nurse specialist (CNS) with specific training and skills in the supervision of epidural infusions (Pain Society 2003). The CNS should be working at, or aspiring to work at, a higher level of practice in the field of acute pain management according to the recommendations for nursing practice in pain management set out by the Pain Society (2003). It is essential that the CNS has a thorough knowledge of:

- the physiology of pain;
- the anatomy of the epidural space;
- the epidural catheter insertion technique;
- the pharmacodynamics and pharmacokinetics of the drugs used in the epidural infusion;
- the delivery device and other equipment used to deliver an epidural infusion;
- the side effects associated with epidural infusion including their recognition and treatment.

ACCOUNTABILITY

Clinical nurse specialists as registered nurses who are accountable for their practice must always act in a manner that promotes and safeguards the interests and well being of patients receiving epidural analgesia. The CNS must also ensure that no action or omission regarding management of epidural infusions is detrimental to the interests, condition or safety of patients. He or she should maintain and improve professional knowledge and competence regarding regional analgesia and acknowledge any limitations in knowledge and/or competence. The CNS has an obligation to decline duties relating to epidural management unless able to perform them in a safe and skilled manner (Nursing and Midwifery Council (NMC), 2004). Competence is described by the NMC (2004) as possessing the skills and abilities required for lawful, safe and effective professional practice without direct supervision.

INFORMATION GIVING

The nurse specialist should be available preoperatively to provide both verbal and written information to patients in a bid to reduce anxiety and pain (Audit Commission, 1998). The material should be accurate, truthful and presented in a way that may be easily understood by patients and in a format appropriate to meet their individual needs (NMC, 2004). An example of useful patient documentation is the RCA and AAGBI (2004) booklet entitled *Epidurals for Pain Relief after Surgery* which can be downloaded from the internet at www.youranaesthetic.info (see Figure 1.1).

Being prepared will help put patients in control and enable them to make informed choices regarding epidural analgesia. The CNS and other members of the multidisciplinary pain management team must remember that it is important to be sensitive to patients' needs and to respect the wishes of those who refuse information (NMC, 2004).

CONFIDENTIALITY

The CNS along with all members of the multidisciplinary pain management team must treat all information about patients as confidential and use it only for the purposes for which it was given. Breaches or improper disclosure of confidential information must be guarded against at all times (NMC, 2004).

CLINICAL ROLE

The CNS has a key clinical role within the pain team for providing evidence based epidural care. His or her responsibilities include at least once daily visits to each patient receiving an epidural infusion in order to assess efficacy in conjunction with the patient and the ward staff. To achieve this there must be documented evidence of an appropriate pain assessment tool in existence, i.e. a verbal or numerical rating scale (Chapter 8). The pain assessment should be performed regularly using the designated tool and scores obtained must be documented on an appropriate monitoring chart. If the patient complains of pain the epidural should be checked to ensure that the infusion is in progress and that the catheter has not become disconnected or dislodged.

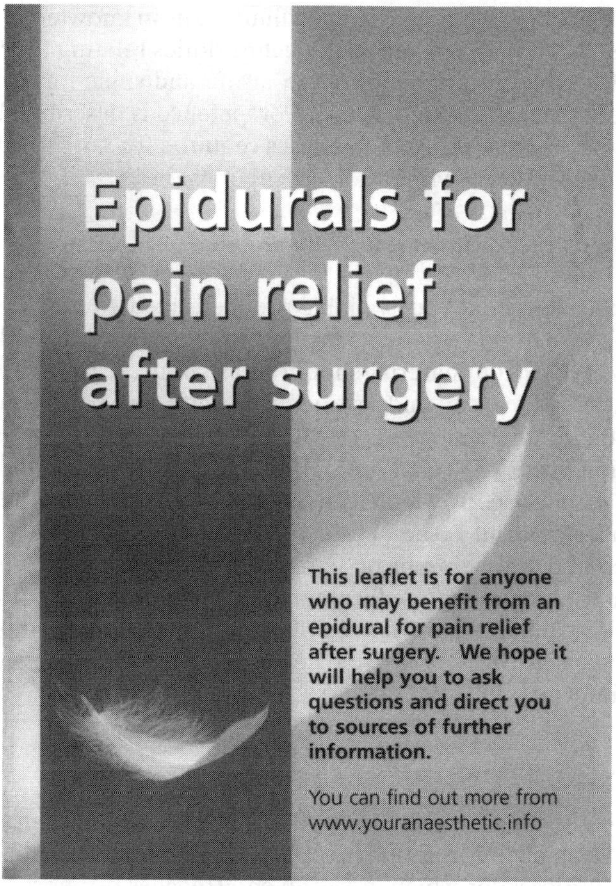

Figure 1.1. Royal College of Anaesthetists patient information booklet *Epidurals for Pain Relief after Surgery*. (Reproduced by permission of the Royal College of Anaesthetists.)

If there is a technical problem with the infusion device or other equipment the CNS should rectify this (Chapter 10). If the equipment is working well but the patient continues to complain of pain, a dermatomal block test should be performed (Chapter 3). If there is insufficient block provided by the infusion, the anaesthetist should be contacted and a prescription obtained for the infusion rate to be adjusted and/or for a bolus dose of epidural solution to be administered via the epidural catheter to the patient. Bolus administration should be undertaken as per the local protocol and with strict monitoring in place (Chapter 10).

It is also important to ensure that adjuvant analgesia is prescribed (Chapter 4), as outlined in the World Health Organisation analgesic ladder, and administered appropriately. It may be necessary to give advice to ward doctors and nurses regarding the importance of regular administration of balanced analgesia alongside the epidural infusion.

The CNS should also assess and advise on the management of any adverse drug reactions or other side effects attributed to the epidural infusion. The charts should be reviewed and the patient questioned in order to establish if the patient has suffered from over-sedation, reduced respiratory function, hypotension, nausea and vomiting, hallucinations, headache, urinary retention, increased motor block or any other associated drug side effects. If any of these problems exists appropriate remedial action must be taken to ensure the patient's safety and comfort (Chapter 10).

The insertion site of the epidural catheter should also be checked for any signs of infection; if there is any redness, swelling or pus evident at the site or if the patient has a pyrexia of unknown origin the epidural infusion should be stopped. The catheter should then be removed as soon as is appropriate (Chapter 9) and the tip of the catheter sent for culture and sensitivity. If necessary, dependent on the laboratory reports, the patient may need a course of appropriate antibiotics.

The CNS should also keep appropriate written records and liaise and work co-operatively with other members of the healthcare team respecting the skills, expertise and contributions of colleagues (NMC, 2004).

RECORD KEEPING

The CNS has a responsibility for record keeping which helps to protect the welfare of patients by promoting:

- high standards of clinical care;
- continuity of care;
- better communication and dissemination of information between members of the interprofessional healthcare team;
- an accurate account of treatment and care planning and delivery;
- the ability to detect problems such as changes in the patient's condition at an early stage (NMC, 2005).

The quality of the records kept reflects the standard of professional practice, therefore good records are the sign of a skilled and safe practitioner. The CNS should keep pain service records for each patient to allow tracking of caseload; they should also make appropriate entries into the multidisciplinary case notes held on the ward or department where the patient is being cared for. The documentation should be legible, factual, consistent and accurate.

They should be written at the time of reviewing the patient or as soon afterwards as possible. Each entry must be signed, dated and timed. Writing should be clear and any alterations, deletions or additions should also be signed with the date and time entered. Abbreviations, jargon, speculation and offensive subjective statements should be avoided (NMC, 2005).

Information technology is being increasingly used within health care as a method of storing patient data. This system has the advantages that notes are easier to read and less bulky; duplication is reduced and access and communication increased across the interprofessional healthcare team. The CNS is professionally accountable for making sure that the system used is robust and secure; the basic principle for computerised records is guided by the Data Protection Act.

The period for which dedicated pain service patient records should be kept will depend on legislation and health service policy statements issued by the Department of Health. Local protocols will provide specific information, but records should be kept for at least eight years for adults and in the case of children at least until the date of their 21st birthday (NMC, 2005).

COMMUNICATION

The CNS is responsible to ensure that effective written and verbal communication within the healthcare team takes place. Good communication allows knowledge, skills and expertise to be shared with other members of the multidisciplinary healthcare team (NMC, 2004).

EDUCATION AND TRAINING

To practise competently the CNS must possess the knowledge, skills, abilities and competence required for lawful, safe and effective practice without direct supervision. The CNS should acknowledge the limits of professional competence and only undertake practice and accept responsibilities for those activities in which he or she is competent. If an aspect of practice is beyond the individual's level of competence or training he or she should obtain help and supervision from a competent practitioner until appropriate knowledge and skills have been acquired (NMC, 2004).

Improvements in epidural education have led to improved pain relief for patients; the CNS is ideally positioned to influence nursing practice relating to epidural management. The CNS is responsible for supporting and teaching pre- and post-registration ward nurses to enable them to provide evidence based pain management for all patients receiving epidural analgesia within their care. They are also responsible for providing education to unqualified nurses who provide general care for patients receiving epidural analgesia.

Finally, the CNS has a responsibility for the education of house officers (and other grades) employed within the anaesthetic department. There should be a formal induction course for those clinicians responsible for supervising patients receiving continuous epidural analgesia.

Education should encompass the theoretical side of epidural management including physiology of pain and pharmacology of epidural drugs and competency based training surrounding safe and effective use of the drug delivery devices (Chapter 11). Additional arrangements for education must be put in place where changes are made to the protocols, equipment or drugs used within the epidural service.

It is essential that the CNS works in collaboration with the training and development department within the trust when devising education and training programmes.

DEVELOPMENT OF A LINK NURSE SCHEME

Development of a link nurse scheme is a useful way of increasing the success of the partnership between the pain team and ward based staff. Link nurses have been recognised as playing a part in improving and maintaining the quality of patient care by disseminating information and research based practice from the pain team to the ward area.

AUDIT AND RESEARCH

The CNS has a responsibility for promoting the participation of acute pain services in local and national audits of epidural analgesia (for further information see Chapter 12). Audit forms part of the process for ensuring that a quality epidural service is being delivered and should examine adherence to monitoring standards, effectiveness of epidural infusions, side effect profiles and other epidural related issues such as patient satisfaction. Examples of appropriate audits are given by the RCA in the audit recipe book (2002). Audit tools should be devised at a local level and care monitored against preset standards. Results of local audits should be disseminated to the anaesthetists and also to ward nursing staff (Chapter 12).

Clinical nurse specialists should actively participate in research projects relating to epidural analgesia and should be involved in maintaining and developing strong links with research institutions. The CNS may also initiate research projects or contribute to departmental projects.

It is vital that the CNS reviews current literature and disseminates this information to ward and departmental nursing staff. CNSs are in a key position to help reduce the perceived theory–practice gap. Practice should be reviewed regularly in light of new research findings and changes made to protocols and practice where appropriate.

MANAGERIAL

The CNS has a responsibility, in association with the consultant anaesthetist, to develop standards of care for epidural practice, local guidelines and protocols in order to maintain a safe environment for the patient. Such protocols, according to the RCA and AAGBI (2004), should describe:

- overall management of patient with epidural infusions;
- instructions for the use of the pump and for troubleshooting;
- description of the drug concentrations used in the hospital;
- instructions for changing epidural solution bags/syringes;
- frequency of observations;
- identification and management of complications;
- management of inadequate analgesia;
- management of accidental catheter disconnection;
- instructions for removal of the epidural catheter;
- management of patients receiving anticoagulants.

Patients receiving epidural infusions must be nursed in a setting which allows close supervision of the patient by appropriately trained staff and where oxygen and resuscitation equipment is available (RCA and AAGBI, 2004). It is the responsibility of the CNS to ensure that these conditions are met.

The CNS also has a responsibility to write business plans in order to ensure continued development of the epidural service in line with changing evidence based practice. Business planning is a continuous process that must be regularly updated; it helps providers to determine local need and commissioners to allocate appropriate funding to secure necessary equipment or staffing in order to sustain or develop the service.

The business case document should put forward the purpose of the epidural service (or a specific part of it) and a vision for the future. It is often useful to start with a SWOT (strengths, weaknesses, opportunities and threats) analysis, which will help to show priorities for the service. The business plan should outline broad aims and objectives, a description of the service at present and of the service required. It should provide information about those people at whom the service is targeted and all of the intended changes will need to be documented. Financial planning is crucial with targets highlighted for income and expenditure. Quality standards should be set along with a plan for staff development to meet the proposed standards. Finally, details of a proposed audit programme to measure standards should be defined.

Although every pain service is different the principles that underpin all epidural services are similar. It is important to include everyone in the business planning who has a stake in the service including existing colleagues, clinicians, professionals allied to medicine, administrative staff, managerial staff, carers and users. Also any external agencies such as appropriate patient groups and local commissioners.

RESPONSIBILITIES OF THE ANAESTHETIC/ RECOVERY NURSE

The anaesthetic and/or recovery nurse has exactly the same responsibilities as those outlined in the next section entitled 'Responsibilities of the registered nurse'. In addition to this he or she is also responsible for maintaining up-to-date records of the patients currently receiving epidural analgesia, the pump being used (i.e. device identification numbers) and the ward area where the patients are residing.

The recovery nurse also has a responsibility to ensure that prior to leaving recovery the patient with an epidural infusion, who has also undergone a general anaesthetic, should be conscious with return of reflexes and should be able to maintain his or her own airway. The respiratory rate and pattern should be adequate, with no concerns regarding central and peripheral perfusion. The patient's blood pressure, pulse and oxygen saturations should have returned to preoperative levels and be stable and adequate analgesia should have been achieved. Attention should be directed to the effects of any residual motor blockade following regional anaesthesia.

The recovery staff should hand over their patient to the ward nurse or escort nurse with all relevant documentation and the patient should be transported back to the ward area with oxygen, suction and monitoring equipment appropriate to the patient's condition.

RESPONSIBILITIES OF THE REGISTERED NURSE

It is the responsibility of every qualified nurse to maintain individual professional knowledge and competence appropriate to the level at which they are practising (NMC, 2004). Epidural infusions should only be utilised in ward areas where they are frequently used so that nurse expertise and patient safety can be maintained (RCA and AAGBI, 2004). Patients receiving continuous epidural analgesia must always (24 hours per day) be under the direct supervision of a nurse or nurses trained in the management of continuous epidural analgesia who are able to be with the patient within seconds of being summoned. If an aspect of practice is beyond the individual's level of competence he or she should obtain help and supervision from the pain team CNS or anaesthetist. The nurse should be aware of contact numbers that can be used to call the pain team CNS or anaesthetist at any time, day or night, for advice regarding epidurals.

The registered nurse should work within local protocols, procedures and guidelines relating to epidural analgesia practice. If at any time these guidance documents cannot be adhered to, the nurse should inform his or her direct line manager outlining the problems.

The nurse has a responsibility to monitor patients receiving epidural analgesia recording the observations set out in Chapter 8. At least two-hourly recordings of temperature, blood pressure, pulse, respiratory rate, sedation scoring and motor block should take place. In order to undertake effective monitoring nurses should receive appropriate education to understand nociceptive pain pathways, the anatomy of the epidural space and catheter insertion techniques. They also need teaching relating to the pharmacology of opioids and local anaesthetics and management of associated adverse drug reactions.

Registered nurses should provide documented evidence of regular pain scoring using an appropriate tool. Documented evidence that any failure of analgesia has been acted upon should also be recorded. The nurse should also ensure balanced analgesia has been prescribed and administer it appropriately.

As well as these observations, pump monitoring should be undertaken ensuring that the device is delivering the correct drugs to the correct patient in the correct doses. This information should be documented on an appropriate dedicated monitoring chart. In order to manipulate the device to check the infusion rates, etc., nurses should undergo specific competency based training on the device being used (Chapter 11).

The registered nurse has a responsibility to check the epidural catheter site at least once per shift while the infusion is in progress and once per day for 48 hours after the epidural catheter has been removed. This check should be carried out to identify any potential problems with local infection at the epidural site, so vigilance for any signs of redness, swelling, soreness or pus is essential. If infection is suspected the catheter should be removed as soon as possible (Chapter 9), the tip sent for culture and sensitivity, the entry site cleaned and re-dressed and the pain team CNS informed.

Any drug incidents that occur should be documented and reported to the registered nurse's direct line manager, the pain team and also the pharmacy department. Any faults with technical equipment should be reported to the pain team and the electrical engineering department so that appropriate remedial action can be taken.

Qualified nurses should also be appropriately trained to remove the epidural catheter once the infusion has been discontinued. Specific information relating to catheter removal can be found in Chapter 9.

Issues relating to confidentiality and record keeping (including electronic records) apply in the same way as set out above for the CNS. All information should be treated as confidential and should not be inappropriately disclosed. Patient records should be kept up to date, with accurate and complete entries that are clearly written, timed and dated (NMC, 2005).

Where appropriate, registered nurses should participate in audit programmes and be prepared to participate in change management practice to ensure evidence based best practice is maintained.

RESPONSIBILITIES OF THE PHARMACIST

The pharmacist has a specific role within the pain team in relation to epidural infusions. They should be invited to participate actively in the production of prescribing guidelines for epidural analgesic drugs, and the co-prescribing of balanced analgesia, an opioid antagonist and antiemetics. They should also be involved in decisions about patient information leaflets regarding epidural infusions that are distributed to patients preoperatively in a bid to ensure that any pharmacological information is accurate and appropriate.

They should regularly monitor prescriptions of epidural solutions where preprinted prescriptions are not utilised and of adjuvant therapies such as antiemetics and opioid antagonists. It is also helpful if a designated pharmacist attends regular pain team link nurse/pharmacist meetings where results of such monitoring can be discussed.

Pharmacists are best placed to devise policies to ensure safe and legal handling, administration and disposal of the controlled drugs utilised within epidural infusions. They should advise on storage arrangements that ensure that the drugs required are purchased and distributed to the designated storage areas of the hospital for the epidural service to run smoothly. They must ensure that if epidural solution is made up in the local pharmacy area of the hospital (rather than being bought from an external supplier) it is prepared aseptically and appropriately labelled and stored within the department.

Consistency of advice and information regarding epidural infusions is essential; the pharmacist plays a pivotal role in communication to pain team, ward nurses and medical staff.

RESPONSIBILITIES OF THE ELECTROBIOMEDICAL ENGINEERING DEPARTMENT

The electrobiomedical engineering (EBME) department is an essential support for an epidural service. Engineers along with members of the pain team and procurement department should be involved in choosing appropriate pump devices to deliver the epidural infusions (for further information see Chapter 5). The equipment chosen should ensure safe and effective utilisation of epidural infusions with the following safety mechanisms: programming in millilitres per hour, rate capping, printable extended history via key stroke logging, locking with restricted access, clear vision of fluids, adjustable pressure limits, bolus administration with restricted access for specialist users and bolus administration by patients. The device chosen should be standardised throughout the institution so that it is familiar to all staff involved in providing or supervising epidural infusions (RCA and AAGBI, 2004). Specific handbooks relating to the device should be available in all areas where the device is used.

The engineering department should configure new pumps with preset parameters for maximum infusion rates and bolus sizes, which should be agreed with the pain team consultant anaesthetist and senior CNS. Pumps should be marked so that it is clear that they should be used exclusively for epidural analgesia and the engineers should be aware of the training programme that is in place for all device users.

There are a number of clear guidance documents that direct the engineering department regarding medical devices including the MDA DB 9801 medical devices and equipment management for hospital and community based organisations, the MDA DB 9801 supplement one which checks and tests for newly delivered medical devices and the Welsh Risk Management Standard 30 Medical equipment and devices.

The engineers are involved in equipment service test procedures or performance verification procedures. The frequency of service can vary between manufacturers and device models, although it is recommended that devices are subject to one annual maintenance service to include a full function and electrical safety test.

If pumps fail, the engineering department should undertake repair work. Formal work instructions follow the manufacturer's guidance, which is obtained from the manufacturer's operating and service instruction manuals. Engineers are responsible for all service and repair records, which are retained on an equipment management database.

RESPONSIBILITIES OF THE HEADS OF NURSING AND CLINICAL MANAGERS

Pain management is recognised as a subspeciality of anaesthesia, therefore financing and organisation of service developments and delivery are the remit of the anaesthetic business managers (AAGBI and Pain Society, 1997).

Managers should ensure adequate resources are available to provide an epidural analgesia service, i.e. funding for appropriate personnel, devices, drugs, sterile products, etc. They also have a responsibility to allow adequate study time for nursing and medical staff to attend epidural analgesia education and pump training sessions.

The managers should assist by putting systems in place to promote health and safety awareness of guidelines, protocols and policies, i.e. a local intranet system where appropriate information can be easily accessed at ward level. There should also be a system in place for professional support and advice for the CNS in pain management and the opportunities for clinical supervision to take place.

REFERENCES

Association of Anaesthetists of Great Britain and Ireland (2001) *Preoperative Assessment: the Role of the Anaesthetist*. London: The Association of Anaesthetists of Great Britain and Ireland.

Association of Anaesthetists of Great Britain and Ireland and the Pain Society (1997) *Provision of Pain Services*. London: Alresford Press.

Audit Commission (1998) *Audit Commission Act*. London: Stationery Office.

Bibby, P. (2001) Introducing ward based epidural pain relief. *Professional Nurse*, **16** (6), 1178–81.

Nursing and Midwifery Council (2004) *Code of Professional Conduct, Standards for Conduct, Performance and Ethics*. London: NMC.

Nursing and Midwifery Council (2005) *Guidelines for Records and Record Keeping*. London: NMC.

Pain Society (in conjunction with the RCA) (2003) *Pain Management Services – Good Practice*. London: RCA.

Royal College of Anaesthetists (2002) *Raising the Standard – A Compendium of Audit Recipes for Continuous Quality Improvement in Anaesthesia*. London: RCA.

Royal College of Anaesthetists and the Association of Anaesthetists of Great Britain and Ireland (2002) *Good Practice: a Guide for Departments of Anaesthesia, Critical Care and Pain Management*, 2nd edn. London: RCA/AAGBI.

Royal College of Anaesthetists and the Association of Anaesthetists of Great Britain and Ireland (2004) *Epidurals for Pain Relief after Surgery*. London: RCA/AAGBI.

Royal College of Anaesthetists, Royal College of Nursing, the Association of Anaesthetists of Great Britain and Ireland, the British Pain Society and the European Society of Regional Anaesthesia and Pain Therapy (2004) *Good Practice in the Management of Continuous Epidural Analgesia in the Hospital Setting*. London: RCA.

Royal College of Surgeons and the Royal College of Anaesthetists (1990) *Pain after Surgery*. Report of a working party of the commission on the provision of surgical services. London: RCSE/RCA.

2

Patient Selection

LYNDA JENKINS

Clinical Nurse Specialist in Pain Management,
Morriston Hospital, Swansea, South Wales

Effective analgesia for postoperative pain relief following major surgery is acknowledged to reduce the symptoms of injury response and improve surgical outcomes. In upper abdominal surgery epidural analgesia is perceived by 80% of UK anaesthetists as the ideal analgesic technique, but many patients who might benefit from this type of analgesic system do not receive it because perceived risks outweigh benefits. This chapter considers the selection of patients who would benefit from epidural analgesia when undergoing major surgery, it reviews the risk–benefit analysis and also considers the issues of informed consent.

PATIENT SELECTION

Patient selection for the placement of an epidural catheter and subsequent delivery of analgesia for pain management should be against a stringent risk–benefit assessment. The anaesthetist undertaking the anaesthetic management should carry out this evaluation.

Epidural analgesia should be a planned procedure with not only the risk–benefit to the patient taken into account, but also the medical and nursing skill mix available to manage the patient pre-, intra- and postoperatively. Time of day will have an impact on management and selection of suitable patients,

Epidural Analgesia in Acute Pain Management. Edited by Carolyn Middleton.
© 2006 by John Wiley & Sons, Ltd.   ISBN 0-470-01964-6

as complex regional techniques are not recommended on patients during late evening and night time surgery.

RISKS OF EPIDURAL ANALGESIA

There are a number of complications that can result from epidural analgesia some of which are of major importance when balancing the need for quality analgesia against potential risk. The formation of acute pain teams is important to enable early recognition and treatment of not only the more common complications, but also for instigating corrective action for the rarer complications to limit or prevent permanent harm (Chapter 10).

NEUROLOGICAL COMPLICATIONS

Serious neurological injury by direct trauma to spinal cord or nerve root occurs very rarely with lumbar epidural analgesia; this is also true of thoracic placements. For patients undergoing major surgery the risk of permanent nerve damage is similar in patients with or without an epidural catheter in place (Kroll *et al.*, 1990). Due to the rarity of permanent neurological damage from epidural analgesia, it is difficult to estimate its incidence, although Dalgren and Tornebrandt (1995) cite the risk as 0.03% and Kane (1981) as 0.006%. The Royal College of Anaesthetists (2004) places the risk as approximately 1 in 100 000.

Epidural catheterisation is most frequently performed in the awake patient who is then able to report to the anaesthetist any pain or paraesthesia while placing the catheter, this helps to avoid the risk of neurological damage (Bromage and Benumof, 1998). However, while this is accepted as best practice, there is still ongoing debate in support of epidural insertion in the anaesthetised patient (Chapter 3) (Fischer, 1998).

Transient Neuropathy

Transient neuropathy with a full recovery occurs more commonly but is still relatively infrequent; a recent prospective multi-centre study involving over 30 000 patients reported only five cases (0.016%) of radiculopathy and over 50% of these patients recovered within three months (Auroy *et al.*, 1997). This result is in line with other previously published large studies on transient neuropathy where Tanaka *et al.* (1993) suggested an incidence of 0.23% and Xie and Liu (1991) reported it to be 0.013%.

Dural Puncture

Inadvertent dural puncture is caused by the epidural needle passing through the epidural space, through the dura mater and into the subarachnoid space causing leakage of cerebrospinal fuild (CSF) from the spinal canal (Chapter 3). This leakage causes a corresponding drop in pressure and allows the subarachnoid membrane, which supplies the nervous system and CSF to the brain, to sag downwards resulting in the development of a post-dural puncture headache. The incidence of dural puncture during epidural insertion occurs in 0.32–1.23% of cases (Scherer *et al.*, 1993; Tanaka *et al.*, 1993; Giebler *et al.*, 1997). The likelihood of developing a post-dural puncture headache varies between 16% and 86% as multiple factors are involved, e.g. needle size and patient age.

Other rare conditions following epidural insertion are neurological deterioration due to subdural haematoma following dural puncture, pneumocephalus, venous air embolism, spinal cord and nerve root compression (Diemunsch *et al.*, 1998; Katz *et al.*, 1990; Mateo *et al.*, 1999). The use of saline instead of air with loss of resistance technique (Chapter 3) may reduce the incidence of many of these problems (Sethna and Berde, 1993; Saberski *et al.*, 1997).

Spinal Haematoma

Puncture of epidural vessels during catheter placement occurs during 3–12% of attempts (Schwander and Bachmann, 1991), but the subsequent development of a spinal haematoma causing neurological damage is a rare but potentially devastating complication of epidural catheter placement. If not detected (Chapter 10) and decompressed early it can result in irreversible paraplegia.

The actual incidence of clinically apparent epidural haematoma is unknown and the reported incidence varies greatly between studies. A review of 850 000 epidural anaesthetics and 650 000 spinal techniques by Tryba (1993) identified only 13 cases of spinal haematoma among the epidural techniques and seven cases of spinal haematoma among the spinal techniques. The calculated incidence for a spinal haematoma based on Tryba's work is reported to be less than 1 in 150 000 for an epidural anaesthetic and less than 1 in 220 000 for a spinal anaesthetic (Tryba 1993). As these estimates represent the upper limit of the 95% confidence interval, the actual frequency may be much less.

Examination of all case reports of spinal haematoma has revealed potential risk factors such as haemostatic abnormality. Vandermeulen *et al.* (1994) reported 61 cases of spinal haematoma associated with epidural or spinal anaesthesia from 18 studies involving 200 000 patients. In 42 of the 61 patients

(68%) there was evidence of haemostatic abnormality and 12 patients had evidence of coagulopathy or thrombocytopenia or were treated with antiplatelet agents, thrombolytics or anticoagulants.

Anticoagulant therapy administration can increase the risk of haematoma and increases in incidence are being reported since the introduction of a newer generation of anticoagulants. This has been partly evident in America where larger doses are used compared with other countries. Development of a haematoma is not just related to insertion but also (of equal importance) to the removal of the epidural catheter in relation to anticoagulant administration (Chapter 9). In Vandermeulen *et al.*'s (1994) study it was reported that 30 patients who developed a haematoma had received either intravenous or subcutaneous unfractionated or low molecular weight heparin and in nearly 50% of cases the spinal haematoma occurred immediately after removal of the epidural catheter (Vandermeulen *et al.*, 1994).

Infection

Any patient with local or systemic infection is potentially at risk of developing neuraxial infection, therefore extreme vigilance must be maintained in the monitoring and detection of epidural infection (Chapter 8). It is generally recommended that patients with untreated bacteraemia should not be candidates for epidural catheterisation unless the benefits outweigh the risks.

Infection can be introduced into the epidural space from:

- an exogenous source – contaminated equipment or drugs;
- an endogenous source – leading to bacteraemia;
- a catheter that may act as a wick – infection tracks down from the entry site on the skin to the epidural space.

Infection can result in either meningitis where the dura is breached or epidural abscess formation leading to spinal cord compression. It is difficult to estimate the incidence of epidural abscess as it is a rare occurrence, but several small-scale studies place it at between 1 in 10000 and 2 in 13000 (Kindler *et al.*, 1996; Rygnestad *et al.*, 1997; Wang *et al.*, 1999). When cord compression does occur if decompression is not performed early, irreversible paraplegia can ensue. The incidence of persistent neurological deficit from an epidural abscess is almost 50%, and this outcome has not improved since the period 1947–74 (Kindler *et al.*, 1996).

The findings of a Danish study suggest that patients who developed an epidural abscess had a longer mean catheterisation time and the majority of the patients were immunocompromised by one or more complicating diseases, e.g. malignancy, diabetes, multiple trauma or chronic obstructive airways disease. This predominance of immunocompromised patients has also been found in previous studies (Kee *et al.*, 1992). In most cases perioperative anti-coagulant therapy was also involved (Wang *et al.*, 1999).

Catheter Migration

After placement of an epidural catheter, it is possible for the tip to migrate into the subarachnoid space (Chapter 3), resulting in a high block or a total spinal anaesthesia with possible neurotoxicity following local anaesthetic delivery. Therefore, careful aspiration to detect the presence of cerebrospinal fluid or a small test dose of local anaesthetic is recommended as a way of providing evidence of catheter migration. However, the increasing use of low dose local anaesthetic–opioid infusions has helped to prevent the above dramatic complication happening. The incidence of intrathecal migration has been reported as 0.15–0.18% (Ready *et al.*, 1991; Schug and Torrie, 1993)

DRUG RELATED RISKS

All drugs infused into the epidural space to provide postoperative analgesia carry the potential for serious adverse effects.

Local Anaesthetic Adverse Effects

Central Nervous System Toxicity

Local anaesthetic cardiovascular and central nervous system toxicity occurs when an inadvertent local anaesthetic overdose is administered into the wrong compartment, i.e. intrathecal space instead of into the epidural space. It can also occur if the local anaesthetic is administered directly into the circulatory system or if incorrect concentration or volume of local anaesthetic is used.

The resulting high plasma concentrations of free local anaesthetic cause central nervous system toxicity (Chapter 4), notably convulsions, and may lead to cardiorespiratory arrest if not detected and treated. Brown *et al.*'s (1995) study of 16 870 patients and Tanaka *et al.*'s (1993) study of 40 010 patients both reported the incidence of central nervous system toxicity in patients receiving bupivacaine to be between 0.01% and 0.12%. Cerebral irritation has been documented in doses as low as 30 mg/hour (Dunne and Knox, 1991), this dose was still considerably higher than the 'optimal' dose of bupivacaine recommended by Curatolo and colleagues (2000) for local anaesthetic–opioid combination. The increasing use of low concentration local anaesthetic–opioid combinations coupled with the use of dedicated infusion pumps, which have the capacity to be rate capped, should help to avoid the incidence of central nervous system toxicity during the administration of continuous infusions in the future.

Motor Blockade

Excessive motor blockade with the increasing use of low concentrations of bupivacaine in controlled infusions is uncommon, occurring in only 3.0% of patients receiving epidural analgesia (Scott *et al.*, 1995). However, if motor blockade does occur (impairing mobilisation) in combination with sensory block, it may contribute to the development of pressure areas on the heels (Punt *et al.*, 1991; Cohen *et al.*, 1992; Smet *et al.*, 1996) and deep venous thrombosis (Wheatley *et al.*, 1991). Persistent or unexplained motor blockade of one or both lower limbs in patients receiving low dose combination local anaesthetic–opioid epidural should always be viewed with suspicion, as stopping the infusion normally results in neurological improvement within two hours. If this does not occur then a high index of suspicion should be given to exclude a spinal haematoma or abscess (Chapter 10).

Hypotension

Local anaesthetics not only provide sensory and motor blockade, they also have variable haemodynamic effects of sympathetic blockade resulting in hypotension and increased fluid requirements. The degree of hypotension depends upon the actual dose; lower concentrations of local anaesthetics cause less effect on blood pressure. The combined results of three studies involving nearly 9000 patients put the incidence of hypotension during epidural infusion of local anaesthetics at 0.7–3% depending upon the concentration used and the criteria for hypotension. The incidence was reported to be less (0.0625–0.25%) with bupivacaine than with other local anaesthetics (de Leon-Casasola *et al.*, 1994; Rygnestad *et al.*, 1997; Tsui *et al.*, 1997). Interestingly, one study assessing the use of patient controlled epidural analgesia (PCEA) gave a 6.8% incidence of hypotension (Liu *et al.*, 1998).

Opioid Related Adverse Effects

Respiratory Depression

Respiratory depression can occur with all spinally administered opioids if these are given in excessive doses. The risk of delayed respiratory depression is greatest with morphine as its hydrophilic structure results in an increased tendency for the drug to remain in the central nervous system, particularly the cerebrospinal fluid. This can result in cephalad migration to the brainstem and prolonged residence in neural tissue (Chapter 4). Fentanyl and diamorphine are more lipophilic and are therefore less likely to cause delayed respiratory depression. The dose of the opioid being administered via continuous infusion is also an important factor (Chapter 5).

The incidence of respiratory depression reported via numerous studies from data collected by acute pain services is between 0.24% and 1.6% and is often also associated with increased sedation. The higher incidence is more representative of the use of epidural morphine infusions (Fuller *et al.*, 1990; Ready *et al.*, 1991; Xie and Liu, 1991; Stuart-Taylor *et al.*, 1992; Leith *et al.*, 1994; Scott *et al.*, 1995; Rygnestad *et al.*, 1997; Burstal *et al.*, 1998). Liu *et al.* (1998) reported that patient controlled epidural analgesia containing fentanyl and local anaesthetic carries an incidence of respiratory depression of 0.3%.

If patients receiving epidural analgesia are appropriately monitored by ward staff (Chapter 8) and supervised by an acute pain team any deterioration in respiratory rate and/or level of consciousness can be detected and correctly managed (Chapter 10). Respiratory depression rates should be no greater than those reported with any other form of opioid analgesia administration (Breivik, 1995).

ADMINISTRATION ERRORS

Human error is the most common reason for administration errors. Occasionally the wrong drug has been administered into the wrong space – sometimes with tragic consequences. Glucose, antibiotics, thiopentone, potassium chloride (resulting in paraplegia) and total parenteral nutrition have all been inadvertently injected (Forestner and Raj, 1975; Cay, 1984; Patel *et al.*, 1984; Shanker *et al.*, 1985; Lin *et al.*, 1986; Kopacz and Slover, 1990; Whiteley and Laurito, 1997; Kulka *et al.*, 1999).

The use of commercially prepared solutions, extreme care with labelling catheters and drugs together with stringent checking procedures and the use of dedicated infusion pumps should help to avoid these problems in the future (Chapter 5).

BENEFITS OF EPIDURAL ANALGESIA

Epidurals are cited as the 'gold standard' analgesia for major abdominal, lower limb, vascular and joint procedures compared with parenteral opioid analgesia. Epidurals have been shown to help reduce postoperative morbidity in high risk patients and to generally improve postoperative outcomes. This is achieved by lowering the incidence of respiratory and cardiovascular complications and decreasing the stress response (Yeager *et al.*, 1987; Liu *et al.*, 1995b).

The reported postoperative outcome benefits of the epidural technique using local anaesthetics, opioids or their combination in 'low risk' patients are not as impressive (Jayr *et al.*, 1993). However, epidurals should not be considered in isolation but as part of the surgical pathway of care. The combination of neuraxial technique and a multimodal approach to aggressive postoperative rehabilitation maximises the physiological effects of the neural blockade on pain, stress responses and organ function. This allows early enteral feeding leading to improved nutrition along with active physiotherapy enabling early mobilisation.

Stress Response

Stimulation of the sympathetic nervous system for a short period of time is the natural response to events such as a painful stimulus, but prolonged activation can cause multiple system dysfunction including cardiovascular, gastrointestinal, respiratory, genitourinary, musculoskeletal and the immune systems (Marieb, 2000). Epidural analgesia is effective in reducing or abolishing the stress response mediators. In high risk surgical patients modifying the stress response may reduce hypermetabolism and increased demands on mass and general physiological reserves, thereby reducing morbidity (Kehlet, 1997).

Respiratory System

In the patient undergoing thoracic or major abdominal surgery, epidural analgesia using local anaesthetic, opioids or their combination has the ability to improve diaphragmatic functioning. It can also significantly reduce the incidence of pulmonary morbidity in those patients at high risk of developing pulmonary complications (Ballantyne *et al.*, 1998). This was demonstrated in a double-blind study in which the effects of parenteral and epidural morphine on early and late pulmonary function were compared in grossly obese patients undergoing gastroplasty for weight reduction. There was a significantly earlier recovery of peak expiratory flow rate, reduced incidence of pulmonary complications such as atelectasis and a shorter hospital stay in the patients receiving epidural analgesia (Rawal *et al.*, 1984).

Coagulation

Epidural local analgesia can reduce the incidence of deep vein thrombosis and pulmonary embolism following surgery. Tuman *et al.* (1991) provided some evidence to show that epidural analgesia (compared with 'on demand' systemic opioids) can improve vascular graft survival in a study of patients with arteriosclerotic vascular disease undergoing aortic bypass surgery. The study concluded that the incidence of thrombotic and cardiovascular events along with local infection complications was significantly reduced in patients receiving epidural analgesia (Tuman *et al.*, 1991).

The beneficial effects on coagulation are achieved by reducing the hypercoagulable state that can ensue following major surgery. In addition, epidural local anaesthetics block sympathetic activity with resultant dilatation of smooth muscle and improved blood flow. Systemic levels of local anaesthetics are also thought to have a direct effect upon platelet aggregation.

Gastrointestinal Function

Epidural local anaesthetics have been shown to reduce the incidence and duration of postoperative ileus (Liu *et al.*, 1995a). Whereas abdominal pain can inhibit intestinal motility, blockade with local anaesthetic of both afferent nociceptive and efferent sympathetic components of the spinal reflex arc can improve bowel motility. Improved gut motility also allows early enteral feeding. This has been shown to reduce the surgical stress response and postoperative septic complications through improved wound healing. To obtain this benefit, epidural local analgesia should be continued for several days, with opioid doses minimised through the use of a multimodal analgesic regimen (Chapter 4).

Cardiovascular System

Thoracic epidural analgesia can play a part in reducing adverse cardiovascular effects in patients with unstable angina and improving myocardial function. (Bloomberg *et al.*, 1989a, 1989b; Koch *et al.*, 1990; Olausson *et al.*, 1997). A recent meta-analysis of 11 randomised controlled studies comprising 1173 patients showed that epidural analgesia with or without opioids for 24 hours after surgery reduced the risk of postoperative myocardial infarction by 40% (Beattie *et al.*, 2001).

INDICATION FOR USE

Patient selection should be based upon the reported benefits and balanced against known complications as shown in Table 2.1 (Dawson, 1995).

PATIENT FACTORS

1. Impaired pulmonary function due to trauma, medical conditions, atelectasis, infection and/or surgical procedure. Patients with poor respiratory reserve may do better with a plain local anaesthetic rather than a combined local anaesthetic–opioid mix with a multimodal regime of paracetamol +/− non-steroidal anti-inflammatory drug (NSAID) adjuvant.
2. History of difficult pain control in previous surgery
3. Impaired cardiovascular function.
4. Surgical procedures on patients with significant co-morbidity in a bid to reduce mortality.
5. Acute ischaemic pain of lower limbs or pre-emptive analgesia for elective amputation.

Table 2.1. Patient selection based on surgical procedure. (From Dawson PJ (1995) *Anaesthesia and Critical Care* **6**: 69–75. Reproduced by permission of Elsevier Ltd)

Benefit exceeds risk	Risk = benefit	Risk exceeds benefit
Thoracic:	Orthopaedic surgery:	Peripheral limb surgery
Thoracoplasty	Total hip replacement	
Pleurectomy	Total knee replacement	
Thoracotomy		
Pleurodesis		Minor abdominal
Pneumonectomy		procedures
Lobectomy	Lower abdominal	Abdominal procedures in
	surgery:	otherwise healthy
		patients
Oesophogastrectomy	Gynaecological	
	Post-caesarean	
	section	
Abdominal aneurysm	Obstetric pain	
Upper abdominal surgery		
Vascular		
Surgery with extensive		
area of dissection:		
Sarcoma in lower limb		
Radical nephrectomy		
Ileal conduit/aortic node		
Colorectal surgery		
Surgical factors		
Scoliotic back surgery		

6. Patients who have experienced difficulties with systemic opioids due to unmanageable side effects (e.g. malignant cancer pain).
7. Chronic non-malignant pain syndrome that may be responsive to a specific intraspinal therapy such as local anaesthetics, clonidine, muscle relaxants, i.e. baclofen or steroids (e.g. neuropathic pain or muscle spasm unresponsive to oral adjuvant therapy).
8. Pain relief in childbirth.

CONTRAINDICATIONS FOR USE

For some patients the risks will outweigh the benefits and epidural analgesia should not be the chosen mode of analgesic delivery system. The common contraindications are presented in Table 2.2.

Table 2.2. Contraindications to epidural analgesia. (From Dawson PJ (1995) *Current Anaethesia and Critical Care* **6**: 69–75. Reproduced by permission of Elseiver Ltd)

Absolute	Relative
Patient refusal	Administration of low molecular weight heparin
	May be administered 2 hours after
Coagulopathy	insertion or removal of catheter
Platelet count <80000	Should be stopped 12 hours before
Warfarinisation	insertion or removal of catheter
Intraoperative heparinisation	
Previous neurological injury at site of insertion	Patients receiving NSAIDs or aspirin should have a formal platelet function test. Bleeding time is inconsistent
Allergy	
	Diabetes, steroids, immunocompromised –
Lack of suitable conditions for insertion	state where there is an increasing risk of infection
Local sepsis	Dural tap; risk of intrathecal spread of epidural infusion
Lack of trained personnel and guidelines and protocols to guide practice	Back pain or previous trauma at the site of epidural insertion
Technical difficulties	Mechanical – technical difficulties in inserting catheter
Hypovolaemia, shock	
Sleep apnoea	
Elevated intracranial pressure	

PATIENT CONSENT

Informed consent is an ethical responsibility to ensure that patients understand the treatment options available. It is not currently a requirement to obtain written consent from the patient prior to insertion of an epidural catheter, verbal consent is sufficient providing there is evidence that appropriate discussion has taken place. The details of this discussion must be documented in the patient's notes or on the anaesthetic record for medicolegal purposes.

The patient should have access to information regarding not only the benefits of epidural analgesia, but also information relating to possible adverse effects. Discussion of possible complications is often avoided because of concerns about causing anxiety, because the time required to impart the information is limited or the practitioner lacks knowledge of the side effects and complications. The anaesthetist and clinical nurse practitioner for the pain team are both ideally placed to visit the patient preoperatively and provide all relevant information both verbally and in written form (Chapter 1). After being given the information the patient needs time to discuss any issues that may be unclear.

REFERENCES

Auroy, Y., Narchi, P., Messiah, A. *et al.* (1997) Serious complications related to regional anaesthesia: results of a prospective survey in France. *Anaesthesiology*, **87**, 479–86.

Ballantyne, J., Carr, D., deFerranti, S. *et al.* (1998) The comparative effects of postoperative analgesic therapies on pulmonary outcome: cumulative meta-analysis of randomised, controlled trials. *Anesthesia & Analgesia*, **86** (3), 598–612.

Beattie, W., Bader, N. and Choi, P. (2001) Epidural analgesia reduces postoperative myocardial infarction: a meta-analysis. *Anesthesia & Analgesia*, **93**, 85–8.

Bloomberg, S., Curelaru, J., Emanuelsson, H. *et al.* (1989a) Thoracic epidural anaesthesia in patients with unstable angina pectoris. *European Heart Journal*, **10**, 473.

Bloomberg, S., Emanuelsson, H. and Rickstein, S. (1989b) Thoracic epidural anaesthesia and central haemo-dynamics in patients with unstable angina pectoris. *Anesthesia & Analgesia*, **69** (5), 558–62.

Breivik, H. (1995) Safe peri-operative spinal and epidural analgesia: importance of drug combinations segmental site of injection, training and monitoring. *Acta Anaesthesiology Scandinavia*, **39**, 869–71.

Bromage, P. and Benumof, J. (1998) Paraplegia following intra-cord injection during attempted epidural anaesthesia under general anaesthesia. *Regional Anaesthesia and Pain Medicine*, **23**, 104–7.

Brown, D., Ransome, D., Hall, J. *et al.* (1995) Regional anaesthesia and local anaesthetic-induced systemic toxicity: seizure frequency and accompanying cardiovascular changes. *Anesthesia & Analgesia*, **81**, 321–8.

Burstal, R., Wegener, F., Hayes, C. and Lantry, G. (1998) Epidural analgesia: prospective audit of 1062 patients. *Anaesthesia and Intensive Care*, **26**, 165–72.

Cay, D. (1984) Accidental epidural thiopentone. *Anaesthesia and Intensive Care*, **12**, 61–3.

Cohen, S., Amar, D., Pantuck, C. *et al.* (1992) Adverse effects of epidural 0.03% bupivacaine during analgesia after caesarean section. *Anesthesia & Analgesia*, **75**, 753–6.

Curatolo, M., Schnider, T., Petersen-Felix, S. *et al.* (2000) A direct search procedure to optimise combinations for epidural bupivacaine, fentanyl and clonidine for postoperative analgesia. *Anaesthesiology*, **92**, 325–37.

Dalgren, N. and Tornebrandt, K. (1995) Neurological complications after anaesthesia. A follow up of 18000 spinal and epidural anaesthetics performed over three years. *Acta Anaesthesiology Scandinavia*, **39**, 872–80.

Dawson, P. (1995) Postoperative epidural analgesia *Current Anaesthesia and Critical Care*, **6**, 69–75.

de Leon-Casasola, O., Parker, B., Lema, K. *et al.* (1994) Postoperative epidural bupivacaine–morphine therapy. Experience with 4227 surgical cancer patients. *Anaesthesiology*, **81**, 368–75.

Diemunsch, P., Balabaud, V., Petiau, C. *et al.* (1998) Bilateral subdural haematoma following epidural anaesthesia. *Canadian Journal Anaesthesia*, **45**, 328–31.

Dunne, N. and Knox, W. (1991) Neurological complications following the use of continuous extradural analgesia with bupivacaine. *British Journal of Anaesthesia*, **66**, 617–19.

Fischer, H. (1998) Regional anaesthesia – before or after general anaesthesia? *Anaesthesia*, **53**, 727–9.

Forestner, J. and Raj, P. (1975) Inadvertent epidural injection of thiopentone: a case report. *Anesthesia & Analgesia*, **54**, 406–7.

Fuller, J., McMorland, G., Douglas, M. and Palmer, L. (1990) Epidural morphine for analgesia after caesarean section: a report of 4880 patients. *Canadian Journal of Anaesthesia*, **37**, 636–40.

Giebler, R., Scherer, R. and Peters, J. (1997) Incidence of neurologic complications related to thoracic epidural catheterisation. *Anaesthesiology*, **86**, 55–63.

Jayr, C., Thomas, H., Rey, A. *et al.* (1993) Postoperative pulmonary complications. Epidural analgesia using bupivacaine and opioids versus parenteral opioids. *Anaesthesiology*, **78**, 666–78.

Kane, R.E. (1981) Neurologic deficits following epidural or spinal anaesthesia. *Anesthesia & Analgesia*, **60**, 150–61.

Katz, Y., Markovits, R. and Roseberg, B. (1990) Pneumoencephalus after inadvertent intrathecal air injection during epidural block. *Anaesthesiology*, **73**, 1277–9.

Kee, W., Jones, M., Thomas, P. and Worth, R. (1992) Extra-dural abscess complicating extra-dural anaesthesia for caesarean section. *British Journal of Anaesthesia*, **69**, 647–52.

Kehlet, H. (1997) Multi-modal approach to control postoperative patho-physiology and rehabilitation. *British Journal of Anaesthesia*, **78** (5), 606–17.

Kindler, C., Seeberger, M., Siegmund, M. and Scheider, M. (1996) Extra-dural abscess complicating lumbar extra-dural anaesthesia and analgesia in an obstetric patient. *Acta Anaesthesiology Scandinavia*, **40**, 858–61.

Koch, M., Bloomberg, S., Emanuelsson, H. *et al.* (1990) Thoracic epidural anaesthesia improves global and regional left ventricular function during stress induced myocardial ischaemia in patients with coronary artery disease. *Anesthesia & Analgesia*, **71**, 625.

Kopacz, D. and Slover, R. (1990) Accidental epidural cephazolin injection: safeguards for patient-controlled analgesia. *Anaesthesiology*, **72**, 944–7.

Kroll, D., Caplan, R. *et al.* (1990) Nerve injury associated with anaesthesia. *Anaesthesiology*, **73** (2), 202–7.

Kulka, P., Stratesteneffen, I., Grunewald, R. and Wiebalck, A. (1999) Inadvertent potassium chloride infusion in an epidural catheter. *Anaesthetist*, **48**, 896–9.

Leith, S., Wheatley, R., Jackson, L. and Hunter, D. (1994) Extra-dural infusion analgesia for postoperative pain relief. *British Journal of Anaesthesia*, **73**, 552–8.

Lin, D., Becker, K. and Shapiro, H. (1986) Neurologic changes following epidural injection of potassium chloride and diazepam: a case report with laboratory correlations. *Anaesthesiology*, **65**, 210–2.

Liu, S., Carpenter, R., Mackey, D. *et al.* (1995a) Effects of peri-operative analgesic technique on rate of recovery after colon surgery. *Anaesthesiology*, **83**, 75.

Liu, S., Carpenter, R. and Neal, J. (1995b) Epidural anaesthesia and analgesia: their role in peri-operative outcome. *Anaesthesiology*, **82**, 1474–506.

Liu, S., Allen, H. and Olsson, G. (1998) Patient-controlled epidural analgesia with bupivacaine and fentanyl on hospital wards: prospective experience with 1,030 surgical patients. *Anaesthesiology*, **88**, 688–95.

Marieb, E. (2000) *Essentials of Human Anatomy and Physiology*. Harlow: Addison Wesley Longman.

Mateo, E., Lopez–Alarcon, M., Moliner, S. *et al.* (1999) Epidural and sub-arachnoidal pneumocephalus after epidural technique. *European Journal of Anaesthesiology*, **16**, 413–7.

Olausson, K., Magnusdottir, H., Lurje, L. *et al.* (1997) Anti-ischemic and anti-anginal effects of thoracic epidural anaesthesia versus those of conventional medical therapy in the treatment of severe refractory unstable angina. *Circulation*, **96**, 2178–82.

Patel, P., Sharif, A. and Farnado, P. (1984) Accidental infusion of total parenteral nutrition solution through an epidural catheter. *Anaesthesia*, **39**, 38–40.

Punt, C., van Neer, P. and de Lange, S. (1991) Pressure sores as a possible complication of epidural analgesia. *Anesthesia & Analgesia*, **73**, 657–9.

Rawal, N., Sjostrand, U., Christoffersson, E. *et al.* (1984) Comparison of intra-muscular and epidural morphine for postoperative analgesia in the grossly obese: influence on postoperative ambulation and pulmonary function. *Anesthesia & Analgesia*, **63**, 583–92.

Ready, L., Loper, K., Neesly, M. and Wild, L. (1991) Postoperative epidural morphine is safe on surgical wards. *Anaesthesiology*, **75**, 452–6.

Royal College of Anaesthetists and Association of Anaesthetists of Great Britain and Ireland (2004) *Epidurals for Pain Relief after Surgery*. London: RCA/AAGBI.

Rygnestad, T., Borchgrevink, P. and Eide, E. (1997) Postoperative epidural infusion of morphine and bupivacaine is safe on surgical wards. Organisation of the treatment, effects and side-effects in 2000 consecutive patients. *Acta Anaesthesiology Scandinavia*, **41**, 868–76.

Saberski, L., Kondamuri, S. and Osinubi, O. (1997) Identification of the epidural space: is loss of resistance to air a safe technique? A review of the complications related to the use of air. *Regional Anaesthesia*, **22**, 3–15.

Scherer, R., Schmutzler, M., Geibler, R. *et al.* (1993) Complications related to thoracic epidural analgesia: a prospective study in 1071 surgical patients. *Acta Anaesthesiology Scandinavia*, **24**, 29–33.

Schug, S. and Torrie, J. (1993) Safety assessment of postoperative pain management by an acute pain service. *Pain*, **55**, 387–91.

Schwander, D. and Bachmann, F. (1991) Heparin and spinal or epidural anaesthesia: decision analysis. *Ann. Fr. Anaesthesia Reanim.*, **10**, 284–96.

Scott, D., Beilby, D. and McClymont, C. (1995) Postoperative analgesia using epidural infusions of fentanyl with bupivacaine. A prospective analysis of 1014 patients. *Anaesthesiology*, **83**, 727–37.

Sethna, N. and Berde, C. (1993) Venous air embolism during identification of the epidural space in children. *Anesthesia & Analgesia*, **76**, 925–7.

Shanker, K., Palkar, N. and Nishkala, R. (1985) Paraplegia following epidural potassium chloride. *Anaesthesia*, **40**, 45–7.

Smet, I., Vercauteren, M., De Jongh, R. *et al.* (1996) Pressure sores as a complication of patient-controlled epidural analgesia after caesarean delivery. Case report. *Regional Anaesthesia*, **21**, 338–40.

Stuart-Taylor, M., Billingham, I., Barrett, R. and Church, J. (1992) Extra-dural diamorphine for postoperative analgesia: audit of a nurse-administered service to 800 patients in a district general hospital. *British Journal of Anaesthesia*, **68**, 429–32.

Tanaka, W., Watanabe, R., Harada, T. and Dan, K. (1993) Extensive application of epidural anesthesia and analgesia in a university hospital: incidence of complications related to technique. *Regional Anaesthesia*, **18**, 34–48.

Tryba, M. (1993) Epidural regional anaesthesia and low molecular heparin: Pro. *Anasthesiol. Intensivmed. Notfallmed. Schmerzther.*, **28**, 179–80.

Tsui, S., Irwin, M., Wong, C. *et al.* (1997) An audit of the safety of an acute pain service. *Anaesthesia*, **52**, 1042–7.

Tuman, J., McCarthy, R., March, R. *et al.* (1991) Effects of epidural anaesthesia and analgesia on coagulation and outcome after major vascular surgery. *Anesthesia & Analgesia*, **73**, 696–704.

Vandermeulen, E., Van Aken, H. and Vermylen, J. (1994) Anticoagulants and spinal-epidural anaesthesia. *Anesthesia & Analgesia*, **79**, 1165–77.

Wang, L., Hauerbert, J. and Schmidt, J. (1999) Incidence of spinal epidural abscess after epidural analgesia: a national 1-year survey. *Anaesthesiology*, **91**, 1928–36.

Wheatley, R., Madej, T., Jackson, IJ. and Hunter, D. (1991) The first year's experience of an acute pain service. *British Journal of Anaesthesia*, **67**, 353–9.

Whiteley, M. and Laurito, C. (1997) Neurologic symptoms after accidental administration of epidural glucose. *Anesthesia & Analgesia*, **84**, 216–7.

Xie, R. and Liu, Y. (1991) Survey of the use of epidural analgesia in China. *Chinese Medical Journal*, **104**, 510–5.

Yeager, M., Glass, D., Neff, R. *et al.* (1987) Epidural anaesthesia and analgesia in high-risk surgical patients *Anaesthesiology*, **66**, 729–36.

3

Insertion and Epidural Catheter Management

CAROLYN MIDDLETON

Clinical Nurse Specialist in Pain Management, Nevill Hall Hospital, Abergavenny, South Wales

This chapter aims to provide a working knowledge of the anatomy of the spine and the epidural space. A description of the epidural catheter insertion technique and the necessary components such as securing devices and an antibacterial filter will be provided. Information regarding dermatomal block testing and an overview of the monitoring that is required to assess a patient receiving an epidural infusion will also be described.

ANATOMY OF THE SPINE

The spinal column extends from the skull to the pelvis and is made up of 26 vertebrae: 7 cervical, 12 thoracic, 5 lumbar, the sacrum (consisting of five vertebrae fused together into one bone which is incapable of movement) and the coccyx. The spinal column naturally bends forming an 'S' shape with a concave curve at the thoracic and sacral levels and a convex curve at the cervical and lumbar levels (Figure 3.1). This curvature increases strength, helps to maintain balance, acts as a shock absorber and protects the spinal column from fracture. In the different regions of the spinal column some of the features of the

Epidural Analgesia in Acute Pain Management. Edited by Carolyn Middleton.
© 2006 by John Wiley & Sons, Ltd. ISBN 0-470-01964-6

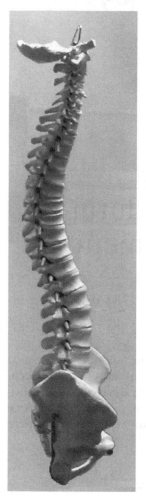

Figure 3.1. Spinal column.

vertebrae change, i.e. they are different shapes and sizes but their make-up remains essentially the same.

Either side of the spinous process of the vertebrae are the transverse processes. Anterior to the spinous process lies the body of the vertebrae, this is the largest part of the vertebrae (smallest in the cervical region and largest in the lumbar region) and linking these structures together are the pedicles and the laminae. Between each vertebra lies the intervertebral disc, which is a protective cushion to stop the vertebrae rubbing against each other.

A spinal nerve passes through the foramen of each vertebra (Figure 3.2). There are 31 pairs of spinal nerves attached to the spinal cord; each is com-

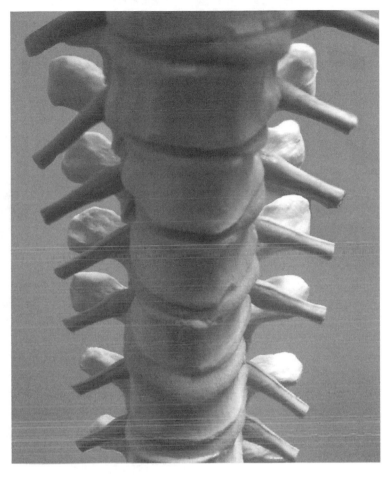

Figure 3.2. Spinal nerves.

posed of an anterior motor root and a posterior sensory root. The nerves are named according to the vertebral level at which they leave the spinal column, i.e. cervical (C), thoracic (T), lumbar (L), sacral (S) and coccygeal (CX). Specific skin areas that are innervated by each of these spinal nerve roots are known as dermatomes (Figure 3.3).

The spinal column provides a protective tunnel for the spinal cord. Surrounding the cord are membranes known as the meninges. There are three layers: the dura mater, which is on the outside; the arachnoid mater, which is the middle layer; and the pia mater, which can be found on the inside. These

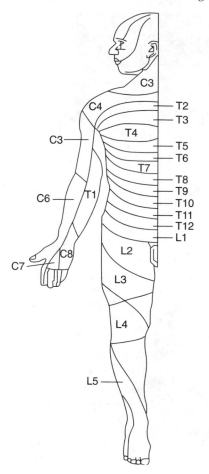

Figure 3.3. Dermatomes.

meninges divide the vertebral canal into three distinctive compartments: the subarachnoid, subdural and epidural spaces.

The epidural space contains extradural fat, blood vessels, lymphatics and nerves. It acts as a cushion between the dura mater and the wall of the vertebral column and it extends from the base of the skull down to the sacrum. The epidural space is in fact only a 'potential' space (particularly in the cervical region) until fluid or air is injected into it. However, in the sacral area where there is no dural sac, the epidural canal can be seen as a more obvious space (Bridenbaugh *et al.*, 1998).

EPIDURAL CATHETER INSERTION

The anaesthetist inserting the epidural catheter should make the final decision regarding patient selection and safety of the procedure (Chapter 2). The patient should be kept informed of what to expect by the anaesthetist at all times. Vital signs such as blood pressure, respiratory rate, sedation score and oxygen saturation levels should be recorded during and after the insertion of the epidural catheter.

Consent

Whenever a procedure is contemplated, informed consent must be obtained unless the patient is deemed to be incapable (Chapter 2). A competent adult has the right under common law to grant or withhold consent to a procedure such as epidural catheter insertion. In order to obtain consent, sufficient information must be given regarding the benefits and risks associated with epidural insertion and possible alternative analgesic techniques that could be employed. The information should be given to the patient in a way that is appropriate to the individual's level of understanding so that an informed choice can be made.

Consent can take several forms such as expressed (either written or verbal) or implied. Expressed consent is required for epidural insertion; this is where the patient confirms their agreement to the procedure in clear explicit terms either in writing or verbally. In the case of verbal consent, all information given to the patient and the patient's agreement to proceed should be documented on the anaesthetic chart or in the case notes. Local policy on invasive techniques will reflect the level of consent required by the patient prior to an epidural catheter being inserted into a patient.

Patient Positioning

There are two possible positions that the patient can adopt for the insertion of an epidural catheter: the lateral position with the knees curled into the abdomen and the chin into the chest; alternatively a seated flexed position where the patient is seated on the edge of the trolley with the feet on a stool and bent forward on to a pillow placed across the knees. The flexion helps with identification of the spinal processes and it also increases separation of the vertebrae to allow maximum widening of the intervertebral spaces and easier access to the epidural space. Once an appropriate position has been adopted and the site of insertion identified the epidural can be performed.

Catheter Insertion

There is some controversy regarding the issue of whether a patient should be awake or asleep during the procedure of inserting an epidural catheter. The debate surrounds the potential for an increased risk of complications in the unconscious patient. There are arguments for the benefits of both asleep and awake insertion procedures, although there is a lack of critical evidence to support one method over the other. The risk–benefit ratio of each procedure should therefore be considered.

The unconscious patient is more relaxed, optimising conditions for insertion of the epidural. There is greater patient acceptance particularly with children and also better conditions for teaching and supervising trainees. The counter-argument is that with a patient who is awake verbal communication can give the first warning signs of nerve contact with the Tuohy needle. Fischer (1998) suggests that there is a perception that nerve damage due to epidural insertion is becoming more common, although there is little published evidence to support this. Any increase in litigation may be due to an increased usage of the procedure or a greater tendency for seeking compensation.

Maximum barrier precautions and observation of universal precautions and product sterility must be employed in order to minimise the risk of infection to the patient during insertion of the epidural catheter (DoH, 2001a). These should include the following procedures.

- Thorough hand washing and the use of gloves. Gloves are not a substitute for hand washing, which should be performed before and immediately after the procedure and before putting on and after removing gloves. Used gloves should be disposed of in an appropriate clinical waste bag (DoH, 2001b). Gloves should be worn to protect hands from contamination from organic matter, microorganisms and toxic substances and to reduce the risk of cross-contamination to both patient and staff (DoH, 2001b). Gloves must conform to the European community standards (CE) and must be of suitable quality and well fitting. For practitioners and/or patients who are sensitive to natural rubber latex, alternative gloves must be made available (Medical Devices Agency (MDA), 1996).
- The wearing of other personal protective equipment (PPE) such as sterile gown, hat and mask, the use of sterile drapes around the insertion site and thorough cleaning of the skin prior to catheter insertion should be implemented. PPE is designed to protect the practitioner from contamination from organic matter, microorganisms and toxic substances and to reduce the risk of cross-contamination to the patient (DoH, 2001a).
- The elements of aseptic technique and protocols for ascertaining product integrity and sterility should be established in organisational policies and procedures (NICE, 2003). The epidural pack and dressings used during this

invasive procedure should be sterile and single use devices must be single use only (MDA, 2000).

- Regulation sharps containers should be used and when three quarters full they should be sealed shut and disposed of by designated personnel (DoH, 2001b). Infection statistics should be audited and documentation retained by each organisation (DoH, 2001a).

Adequate skin preparation is essential if extrinsic mechanisms of infection are to be reduced as colonisation of bacteria and subsequent migration of this bacterium along the catheter into the epidural space is known to be a cause of epidural space infection. Local policies and preferences will vary and determine solutions for skin preparation. The use of chlorhexidine, povidone iodine or other alcohol based solution has been shown to significantly reduce the incidence of catheter related bacteraemia when used for cutaneous disinfection before insertion and for post-insertion site care (Mann *et al.*, 2001). Patient sensitivities should be established prior to skin cleaning procedures being undertaken. Once the skin has been prepared, the solution should be allowed to dry before insertion of any needle.

Owing to the risks of hospital acquired infection, advice should be obtained from a bacteriologist about the need for a hospital policy on antibiotic prophylaxis. This should include management of patients at particular risk of infection such as those with diabetes, on steroid therapy or immunosuppressed (Royal College of Anaesthetists *et al.*, 2004).

The height of epidural insertion is dependent on where the analgesic effect is desired. The epidural should be positioned appropriately so that the dermatomal extent of the block matches exactly the dermatomal extent of the surgery.

Local anaesthetic is injected into the skin and subcutaneous layers at the site of the epidural. A Tuohy needle is then passed using either a midline or paramedian approach (Figure 3.4).

Tuohy needles are widely used throughout the world; their design makes them less likely than the original 'open ended' sharp needles to puncture blood vessels or the dura. The rounded angled tipped Tuohy needle has graduations in centimetres to allow the operating practitioner to see the depth of insertion. The needle is gradually advanced so that it passes through the ligamentum flavum and into the epidural space. A syringe is attached to the end of the needle and the clinician feels for a loss of resistance to air or saline when pressure is applied to the plunger of the syringe. This loss of resistance means that the needle has entered the epidural space (Figure 3.5).

Once the epidural space has been positively identified, the rounded angled tip of the Tuohy needle allows the in-dwelling epidural catheter to be passed through the needle into the space (Figure 3.6). The needle wall is so thin that it will admit a catheter of reasonable size; the needles are available in 16g,

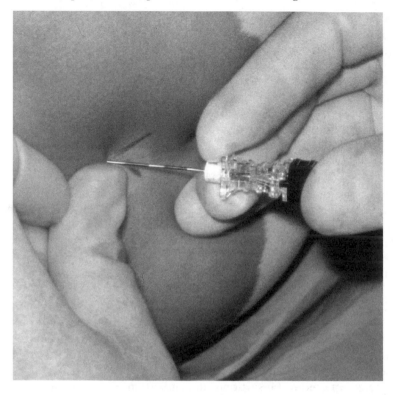

Figure 3.4. Advancement of the Tuohy needle. (Reproduced by permission of B-Braun Medical Ltd.)

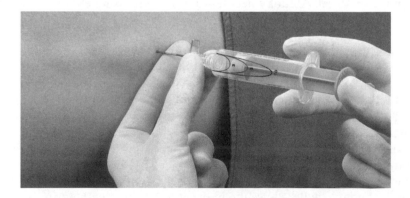

Figure 3.5. Loss of resistance identifies the epidural space. (Reproduced by permission of B-Braun Medical Ltd.)

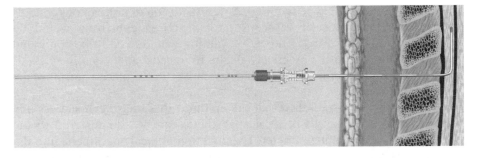

Figure 3.6. Positioning of the catheter in the epidural space. (Reproduced by permission of B-Braun Medical Ltd.)

17 g and 18 g diameter. The catheter should be reasonably rigid to prevent kinking during insertion.

Once the epidural catheter has been positioned, the needle is withdrawn and the catheter length adjusted so that approximately 4–5 cm of catheter are left in the space, this can be assessed by the marked graduations on the catheter. Both the height of the insertion of the epidural (e.g. L2–L3), the depth to the epidural space (e.g. 4 cm) and the length of catheter left in the epidural space (e.g. 5 cm) should be recorded in the patient's notes to act as a reference point for staff when checking the catheter position postoperatively.

Testing for Level of Block

Once the epidural catheter is anticipated to be in place, it is important to verify its location. The catheter should be aspirated to exclude accidental insertion into an epidural vein, if blood is obtained the epidural must be re-positioned. Blood is more easily aspirated through a multi-holed catheter so that in the event of accidental intravascular catheter placement the risk of intravenous injection is reduced (Paech, 2000). If no blood is obtained then a small amount of saline or local anaesthetic should be injected to ensure that the catheter is patent and has not kinked within the epidural space. It is also essential to confirm that the Tuohy needle has not inadvertently punctured the dura – this complication is easily recognised by the immediate loss of cerebrospinal fluid (CSF) through the epidural needle. If the dura is compromised the small test dose of local anaesthetic would be delivered intrathecally and would have a profound effect. If relatively large amounts of opioids and local anaesthetics are administered directly into the CSF a 'total spinal' is observed causing total vasodilation resulting in severe hypotension, a drastic reduction in cardiac output and patient collapse. The patient is likely to suffer respiratory and possibly cardiac arrest. The airway would need to be secured and ventilation with 100% oxygen would be required. A rapid infusion of intravenous colloids and the administration of vasoconstrictors such as ephedrine would be required to increase cardiac output. Ventilation would need to be continued for several hours until the effects begin to recede and consciousness is recovered. The epidural catheter that is inadvertently placed intrathecally must be removed.

Once it has been established that the epidural space has been successfully located, appropriate doses of local anaesthetic can be administered to the patient via the in-dwelling catheter. The insertion of local anaesthetic into the epidural space causes a block of sensory, motor or autonomic nerve roots. A delta and C fibres are nerve fibres responsible for conducting painful stimuli; these fibres are known as nociceptors (Chapter 4). The same fibres also convey information relating to temperature, therefore bathing these fibres with local anaesthetic blocks their ability to conduct both pain and temperature transmission. Checking for a response from the patient to a cold stimulus applied to the skin (such as ice or ethyl chloride) can identify the level and intensity of the nerve block obtained by the local anaesthetic. In dermatomal areas where the patient cannot identify the cold stimulus the nerve roots have been successfully blocked; nerves supplying dermatomal skin areas that continue to be sensitive to cold have not been adequately blocked by the anaesthetic. Testing not only informs the clinician about distribution and quality of the block, but it can also help identify any developing complications such as haematoma.

A unilateral block occurs when analgesia is not provided equally to both sides of the body within the targeted dermatomal areas. This type of block may be associated with poor positioning of the epidural catheter and is particularly associated with the type of catheter which has a terminal eye rather than a closed round-ended tip multi-holed catheter. It is possible for a catheter with only one tip hole to become embedded in the sidewall of the epidural space giving a dense unilateral block effect. Pulling the catheter back a centimetre can sometimes rectify this problem. Clot obstruction can also occur, occluding the tip of the epidural catheter; it is unlikely that this problem can be rectified by moving the epidural catheter position.

There is empirical evidence to suggest that both posture and gravity directly affect the spread of an epidural block. This phenomenon can be effectively utilised in clinical practice by turning the patient on to the side where the block is less dense in a bid to increase the amount of local anaesthetic in that area, increase the block and therefore the analgesic effect in that dermatomal region. Finally, because there is more epidural fat in the lumbar region than in the thoracic area and virtually no epidural fat at all at the cervical level, this can lead to enhanced spread of local anaesthetics at the thoracic level, which can be reduced by a decrease in quantity of local anaesthetic injected (Igarashi *et al.*, 1998).

An increasing amount of motor weakness usually implies one of three occurrences.

1. Excessive epidural drug administration. This can be rectified by a reduction in rate of administration of epidural solution.
2. Dural penetration of the epidural catheter due to migration intrathecally some time after insertion. If this occurs the catheter should be removed.
3. The development of an epidural haematoma or abscess. Haematoma and epidural abscess are classified by extreme loss of motor power and often accompanied by back pain at the site of epidural catheter insertion (Chadwick and Bonica, 1995). Although very rare, if either of these complications is suspected immediate medical attention should be sought as both conditions have the potential for catastrophic effects. Where haematoma is suspected, an MRI scan should be ordered to confirm the diagnosis and immediate treatment of surgical decompression and debridement initiated (Chapter 10).

Securing the Epidural Catheter

The epidural catheter must be effectively secured in place; an epidural that 'falls out' means suboptimal pain relief for the patient. It is paramount that every effort is made to preserve a good working epidural. For this purpose there are many dedicated fixative devices available; some are simple adhesive dressings, others are more complex catheter clamps. There are several important factors to be taken into consideration when choosing a fixative device. First, ease of application of the device. The device should be adhesive to allow firm anchorage of the catheter, however, it should be noted that securing an epidural catheter at its point of entry into the skin does not prevent movement of the catheter relative to the epidural space. For example, if the catheter is inserted in an obese patient in a prone position, it is likely to retract somewhat when the patient adopts a sitting position.

Secondly, the dressing should be occlusive in nature to allow observation and palpation of the catheter exit site for symptoms of local or systemic infection (Chapter 11) (DoH, 2001a). The dressing should prevent build-up of exudates to reduce the risk of microbial contamination and should allow the maintenance of asepsis and provide a barrier to minimise the risk of infection for a minimum of seven days, therefore it is also important that the integrity of the dressing edges is maintained (NICE, 2003). The dressing should not be changed within this period unless it becomes dislodged or direct access to the entry site of the catheter is required. If the site does require re-dressing, a strict aseptic technique must be employed. Occlusive dressings also allow inspection of catheter distance markings without disturbing the dressing. Finally, cost implications and local policy and preferences should be considered when choosing fixation devices and dressings.

Once the catheter is secured at the entry site, the remainder of the catheter should be adhered using hypoallergenic tape to the patient's back then over their shoulder to the point where the antibacterial filter is situated.

Antibacterial Filter

A 'Luer' connector is attached to the end of the epidural catheter and then an antibacterial filter should be attached. The aim of this filter is to minimise the risks of intraluminar bacterial contamination by excluding bacteria and microscopic debris from the epidural and preventing potential development of an epidural abscess (Figure 3.6). The filter should be transparent to allow visual monitoring of filtration. Care should be taken to ensure that the filter does not cause a pressure sore. Many filters are manufactured in the shape of a flat disc specifically to enhance patient comfort and some have self-adhesive devices to hold the filter in place (Figure 3.7). Regardless of the profile there should be regular assessment of the skin under the filter.

There is little good quality evidence to guide practice regarding the changing of the antibacterial filters or epidural administration sets, therefore practice should be guided by the manufacturer's instructions, and local policy. It is generally accepted that filters should not be changed as the risk of contamination is increased.

PATIENT MONITORING

The general principles of observation monitoring pertinent to epidural analgesia will be discussed in Chapter 8, however the important issues relating to epidural insertion will be highlighted here. Local policy will determine both the nature and frequency of vital patient observations and a protocol for monitoring should be in place. The protocol should set out pre-agreed standards and should provide instruction regarding actions to be taken should deviation from these standards be detected.

It may be appropriate to record the observations on a dedicated epidural monitoring chart. It is useful to include pre-epidural observation values for the patient within the dedicated document; this allows comparison of both pre- and postepidural insertion recordings.

Blood Pressure

Hypotension is the most common side effect of epidural analgesia (Berkowitz, 1997). Vasodilatation may occur directly related to sympathetic blockade. However, when hypotension does occur the aetiology should be determined.

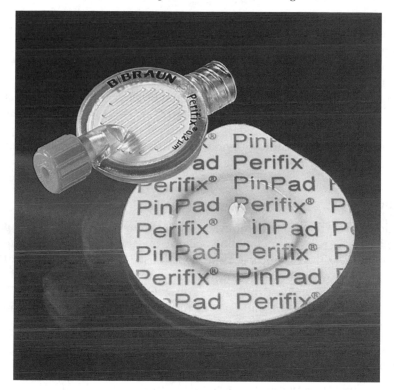

Figure 3.7. Antibacterial filter. (Reproduced by permission of B-Braun Medical Ltd.)

A falling blood pressure associated with an increase in pulse rate, decreasing urine output, loss of skin turgor and a dry mouth indicates dehydration and fluid replacement should be considered. Occasionally vasopressors may be clinically indicated to support the blood pressure. If hypovolaemia is not suspected, then it may be appropriate to reduce the rate of the epidural infusion (Chapter 10).

Respiratory Rate

Absorption of opioids into the circulatory system is detected by specific receptors known as chemoreceptors. These chemoreceptors are ultimately responsible for the homeostasis of both oxygen and carbon dioxide levels in the blood and for relaying vital information to the respiratory centre in the brain stem regarding respiratory activity. Opioid analgesia can have a direct effect on these chemoreceptors resulting in a reduction in respiratory drive and the occurrence of respiratory depression (Richardson, 2003).

Respiratory rate is a key indicator of clinical respiratory depression and respirations should be counted in the unstimulated patient; a rate of less than 12 breaths per minute is deemed to be below the norm for an adult. A respiratory rate of less than eight per minute is considered as a key indicator for respiratory depression. Where respiratory depression does occur an opioid antagonist such as Narcan (naloxone) should be prescribed and administered incrementally by appropriately trained staff. This will reverse the respiratory depressive effects of the opioid in the epidural cocktail. It may be appropriate to continue the epidural with only local anaesthetic being administered to prevent any further respiratory depression occurring.

Sedation Scoring

Sedation scoring is used as an indicator of declining sedation level and potential reduction in respiratory function because excessive sedation enhances respiratory depression. A typical scoring system used is 0 = awake and alert, 1 = occasionally drowsy but easily rousable, 2 = mostly sleeping but easily rousable and 3 = somnolent or difficult to rouse. Opioid dose can be adjusted in light of the sedation score and once again it may be appropriate to continue with a local anaesthetic only epidural infusion.

Oxygen Saturations

Normal cellular function requires adequate oxygen and this depends directly on adequate ventilation, gas exchange and circulatory distribution. Pulse oximetry estimates the amount of oxygen carried on the haemoglobin molecule and therefore makes a contribution to the process of respiratory assessment (Place, 2000). It is a simple procedure that can give continuous recordings, is non-invasive, acceptable to the patient, gives immediate results and allows rapid evaluation of patient response to clinical interventions. Pulse oximetry should, however, only be used as one part of the respiratory status assessment of a patient as this type of monitor relies on translucence of the body at the point of measurement and anything that impedes this will reduce accuracy (Chapter 8).

Pain Assessment

A validated pain assessment tool should be utilised always assessing pain on movement (Chapter 8). Whenever possible this assessment should be done in conjunction with the patient as a more accurate assessment of efficacy of the epidural will be obtained when feedback from the patient is gained. An example of tools that can be used for assessing acute pain in conscious patients who are able to communicate is a visual analogue scale (VAS) using a 10 cm line with endpoints ranging from 'no pain' to 'worst pain imaginable'. Patients are asked to score their pain at an appropriate place along the line, which best represents the intensity of their pain at that time. An alternative is a verbal/numerical rating scale (VNRS), which is a scoring system where numerical values or verbal descriptor of pain intensity are measured. An example is 0 = no pain, 1 = mild pain, 2 = moderate pain and 3 = severe pain on movement.

INTRAVENOUS ACCESS

Prior to insertion of the epidural catheter the patient should have an intravenous cannula inserted. This should remain in place for a minimum of six hours following the removal of the epidural catheter if lipid soluble opioids have been used in the infusion and for 24 hours if lipid insoluble opioids are utilised. Intravenous access is required for immediate administration of naloxone (Narcan), the opioid antagonist, in case of respiratory depression occurring.

URINARY CATHETERISATION

Urinary retention associated with epidurals is caused by inhibition of sacral parasympathetic nervous system outflow causing detrusor muscle relaxation and an increase in maximal bladder capacity. Therefore, urinary catheterisation is recommended for patients receiving epidural analgesia.

REFERENCES

Berkowitz, C. (1997) Epidural pain control: your job too. *Registered Nurse*, **608** (22).

Bridenbaugh, P., Greene, N. and Brull, S. (1998) Spinal (subarachnoid) neural blockade. In: Cousins, M. and Bridenbaugh, P. (eds). *Neural Blockade in Clinical Anaesthesia and Management of Pain*. Philadelphia: Lippincott.

Chadwick, H. and Bonica, J. (1995) Complications of regional anaesthesia. In: Bonica, J. and McDonald, J. (eds). *Principles and Practice of Obstetric Analgesia and Anaesthesia*, 2nd edn. Baltimore: Williams & Wilkins, 538–72.

DoH (2001a) Guidelines for preventing infections associated with the insertion and maintenance of central venous catheters. *Journal of Hospital Infection*, **47** (suppl), S47–S67.

DoH (2001b) Standard principles for preventing hospital acquired infections. *Journal of Hospital Infection*, **47** (suppl), S21–S37.

Fischer, H. (1998) Editorial: Regional anaesthesia – before or after general anaesthesia? *Anaesthesia*, **53**, 727–9.

Igarashi, T., Hirabayashi, Y., Shimizu, R. *et al.* (1998) Thoracic and lumbar extradural structure examined by extra-duroscope. *British Journal of Anaesthesia*, **81**, 121–5.

Mann, T., Orlikowski, C., Gurrin, L. and Keil, A. (2001) The effect of the biopatch, a chlorhexidine impregnated dressing, on bacterial colonization of epidural catheter exit sites. *Anaesthesia and Intensive Care*, **29**, 600–3.

MDA (1996) *Sterilisation, Disinfection and Cleaning of Medical Equipment: Guidance on Decontamination from the Medical Advisory Committee to the DoH*. London: DoH.

MDA (2000) *Single Use Medical Devices: Implications and Consequences of Reuse*. DB 04. London: DoH.

NICE (2003) *Infection Control: Prevention of Healthcare Associated Infection in Primary and Community Care (Clinical Guidelines 2)*. London: NICE.

Paech, M. (2000) Regional analgesia and anaesthesia. In Russell, R. (ed.). *Anaesthesia for Obstetrics and Gynaecology*. London: BMJ Publishing Group.

Place, B. (2000) Pulse oximetry: benefits and limitations. *Nursing Times*, **96** (26), 42.

Richardson, M. (2003) Physiology for practice: the mechanisms controlling respiration. *Nursing Times*, **99** (41), 48–50.

Royal College of Anaesthetists, Royal College of Nursing, the Association of Anaesthetists of Great Britain and Ireland, the British Pain Society and the European Society of Regional Anaesthesia and Pain Therapy (2004) *Good Practice in the Management of Continuous Epidural Analgesia in the Hospital Setting*. London: RCA.

4

Physiology of Pain, Pharmacodynamics and Pharmacokinetics of Local Anaesthetic and Opioid Drugs

CAROLYN MIDDLETON

Clinical Nurse Specialist in Pain Management, Nevill Hall Hospital, Abergavenny, South Wales

The aim of this chapter is to provide healthcare professionals with an overview of the physiology of acute pain and also of the pharmacodynamics and pharmacokinetics of local anaesthetics and opioid analgesic drugs. These two classes of drugs are those most commonly used to provide epidural analgesia to those patients who have undergone major surgery or suffered severe trauma.

PHYSIOLOGY OF ACUTE PAIN

Nociceptors are the receptors responsible for the detection of pain; they are nerve endings, which are located in abundance in the skin, joint capsules, periostea of bones, around the walls of blood vessels and in fewer numbers in the visceral organs. When tissue damage occurs an inflammatory cascade

Epidural Analgesia in Acute Pain Management. Edited by Carolyn Middleton.
© 2006 by John Wiley & Sons, Ltd.   ISBN 0-470-01964-6

begins which starts with enzymes being released from the damaged cells. These enzymes act as chemical irritants and sensitise or irritate the nociceptors causing a pain impulse to be transmitted.

There are different types of nerve fibres, two of which are nociceptive: C fibres which are small and unprotected by myelin and A delta fibres which are slightly larger fibres with a thin layer of protective myelin sheath around them. Myelin is a lipoprotein insulating material that increases the efficiency of transmission of impulses. The impulses travel from one node of Ranvier to another on the myelin sheath jumping over areas of the nerve fibre. The A delta fibres are responsible for the sharp immediate pain felt following the tissue damage (because the myelin increases the conduction speed of the nerve fibre) and the C fibres (which have a slightly slower conduction time as they have no myelin sheath) are responsible for ongoing slower pain transmission. These C fibres continue to be stimulated and fire discharges for a period of time after the removal of the stimulus.

The conduction of pain information relies on action potentials (explosions of electrical activity) taking place in the nerve fibres. An action potential or electrical activity within a nerve cell is caused by an exchange of ions across the neuronal membrane. The inside of a neurone has a negative charge compared with the outside and the nerve cell membrane in its unstimulated state is very much more permeable to potassium ions than it is to sodium ions. When a pain stimulus causes the nerve cell's sodium channels to open there is a rush of sodium ions from the extracellular fluid outside the nerve cell into the intracellular fluid (inside the cell). As sodium has a positive charge attached to it, after the influx of sodium the nerve cell becomes positively charged and depolarises. Once the neurone is depolarised the potassium channels open and potassium ions rush out to the extracellular fluid reversing the depolarisation. The sodium channels close and repolarisation occurs. This all takes place within a millisecond.

An action potential at any one point on an excitable nerve cell membrane will result in excitability of adjoining portions of the membrane, hence the action potential can travel along orders of nerves.

The pain message is transmitted via the afferent pathway along the first order of neurones from the nociceptors in the periphery to the dorsal horn in the spinal column where the A delta and the C nociceptive fibres terminate in the superficial laminae. There is a mechanism described by Melzack and Wall (1965) as the pain gate, which is located in the dorsal horn. This 'gate' is capable of modifying or even inhibiting upward transmission of pain impulses if the large well myelinated non-pain carrying nerve fibres A alpha and A beta are stimulated to a greater extent than the A delta and C nociceptive fibres.

From the dorsal horn the nociceptive information crosses over to the opposite side of the spinal cord and continues travelling via the ascending spinothalamic tract to the thalamus; this is known as the second order of neurones. It then travels via the third order of neurones out to the sensory cortex in the brain where pain is perceived and localised to the specific area of the body where the tissue damaged occurred. At this point the pain becomes a conscious experience. Some nociceptive information travels from the thalamus to the limbic system and emotional responses to the pain ensue.

At each stage in the ascending pathway where nerve fibres meet other nerve fibres (or other structures such as muscles) there is a synaptic cleft, a fluid filled compartment. A single nerve cell may make multiple connections with surrounding nerves via dendrites. The presynaptic action potential from activated nerves sends out neurotransmitters (chemical messengers) from the nerve ending across the synapse to bind with receptors on the postsynaptic nerve ending. These neurotransmitters not only bind with the postsynaptic receptors but also produce an action potential, which allows the nociceptive information to continue on its journey through the central nervous system. The chemicals are only stored presynaptically, therefore impulses are able to be conducted across the synapse in one direction only. The more synaptic clefts that have to be crossed the slower the transmission of the nerve impulse.

From the cerebral cortex the descending pathway is activated and a message travels via the efferent nerve pathway back to the periphery instructing the body to move the affected part away from the source of the pain. The descending pathway includes the cerebral cortex, thalamus and the brainstem. Peri-aqueductal grey matter stimulation initiates the release of inhibitory neurotransmitters (naturally occurring painkillers) such as endorphins, serotonin, 5-HT and gamma aminobutyric acid (GABA) which have opioid-like activity. These endorphins bind with receptor sites and help to modulate or reduce the afferent neurotransmitter activity at the synapse and in doing so reduce the pain experience. These opioid receptors are predominantly found in the central nervous system with approximately 75% of the receptors in the spinal column, 20% in the brain and just 5% in the periphery.

DRUGS USED IN EPIDURAL INFUSIONS

The two classes of drugs that are most commonly used to provide epidural analgesia are local anaesthetics and opioids. These drugs can be given either as single agents or as a 'cocktail' in order to produce a synergistic effect and to reduce the dosages of the single components required.

Drugs for epidural infusions should be aseptically prepared and supplied in clearly identifiable containers. In order to maintain sterility and to reduce the risk of error it is preferable that the solutions are prepared in a central unit (or purchased ready mixed from manufacturers) and not made up by staff in clinical areas (Royal College of Anaesthetists (RCA) and Pain Society, 2003).

All epidural solutions must be clearly labelled distinguishing them from other types of infusion solutions.

The solution (if it contains an opioid) should be stored according to the Control of Drugs Regulations. All epidural solutions should be stored separately from any intravenous fluids so that the local anaesthetic cocktails can never inadvertently be used intravenously. It is advisable on health and safety grounds to have a dedicated control drugs cupboard specifically for the safe storage of epidural solution.

There should be a strict limitation on the number of drugs and the concentrations of these drugs available for epidural infusion use within each hospital (RCA *et al.*, 2004). The drugs and concentrations should be described clearly in hospital protocols or guidelines. Variation from these protocols should occur only in exceptional circumstances and with the agreement of a member of the pain team and/or consultant anaesthetist responsible for pain management.

LOCAL ANAESTHETIC DRUGS

Local anaesthetic drugs are chemical compounds whose primary pharmacological activity involves blocking the conduction process in the peripheral nerves. Like many early therapeutic agents, the first local anaesthetic cocaine was identified in 1884. It was a naturally occurring substance isolated from the 'erythroxylon coca' plant and belongs to the ester group of local anaesthetics. In 1943 lignocaine was synthesised and along with bupivacaine remains the most commonly used local anaesthetic agent in the UK. These substances are known as amide local anaesthetics, they are more stable in solution than the ester agents and do not share the central nervous system excitatory effects. They are therefore less likely to provoke allergic reactions.

Pharmacodynamics of Local Anaesthetics

The conduction of nerve impulses along nerve fibres is related to changes in the electrical gradient across the nerve membrane and movement of predominantly sodium ions (but also potassium ions) from intracellular to extracellular fluid and vice versa. Local anaesthetics work by reversibly blocking specific areas of the nerve cell membrane known as sodium channels. Local anaesthetic agents contain a mixture of ionised and un-ionised particles which, when injected into body tissues, make more un-ionised particles available, which are lipid soluble and able to penetrate the nerve cell membrane. Once inside the nerve cell they become re-ionised and move into and block sodium channels preventing movement of sodium ions across the neuronal membrane. Once the channel is blocked the action potential and therefore nerve conduction are also blocked.

With an epidural infusion the local anaesthetic is injected into the epidural space. A delay in onset of analgesia then occurs because the local anaesthetic needs to spread and diffuse from the epidural space to the spinal nerves. Initially the drug diffuses through the thin layers of dura and arachnoid mater where anterior and posterior spinal nerve roots join to form the spinal nerve (Chapter 3).

The local anaesthetic also diffuses through the dura into the cerebrospinal fluid (CSF) and penetrates the spinal cord. Some of the drug also gains access to the spinal cord via the segmental blood supply. As sensory areas of the spinal cord tend to be more peripheral than motor areas these are affected by local anaesthetic more rapidly and more profoundly. Also the sympathetic small unmyelinated pain impulse carrying nerve fibres, A delta and C fibres, are more rapidly affected and to a greater degree than the larger myelinated A alpha and A beta nerve fibres.

The quality, extent and duration of the epidural nerve blockade can be unpredictable. Local anaesthetic needs to be injected into an area of the epidural space near to where the block is intended, i.e. for an upper abdominal incision or for fractured ribs the epidural catheter entry site should be in the thoracic region, whereas for orthopaedic lower limb surgery a lumbar epidural would be appropriate. An increased volume of local anaesthetic will result in a greater spread of solution within the epidural space and therefore a greater area of block. An increased concentration of local anaesthetic will result in a greater intensity of the block. The integrity of the central nervous system will also have an effect on both spread and intensity of the block.

Pharmacokinetics of Local Anaesthetics

Local anaesthetics can be classified into two groups: amides and esters (Table 4.1). The ester local anaesthetics, such as cocaine, procaine and chlorprocaine, are rapidly metabolised by esterases in plasma and in the liver, therefore systemic toxicity is rare. However, they are pharmaceutically unstable and cause a high incidence of allergic reactions.

Amides such as lignocaine, bupivacaine, ropivacaine and levo-bupivacaine are metabolised more slowly by the liver. They are widely used for epidural

Table 4.1. Classification of local anaesthetics

Amides	Esters
Articaine	Benzocaine
Bupivacaine	Cocaine
Lidocaine	Procaine
Mepivacaine	
Prilocaine	

infusions and have a far lower incidence of allergy than the ester group. Lignocaine has a fast onset and short duration of action; bupivacaine has a slower onset but longer duration of action with less associated motor blockade.

Adverse Effects of Local Anaesthetics

Local anaesthetic has a vasodilating effect, which can potentially cause some degree of hypotension. Using a more dilute local anaesthetic solution or reducing the amount of solution infused may reduce this problem.

Motor blockade is an undesirable side effect that varies in intensity from heavy legs to complete motor blockade. The larger myelinated A alpha and A beta nerve fibres are more difficult to block with local anaesthetic than the smaller less well protected pain carrying A delta and C fibres. It is easy therefore to reverse the degree of motor block by either decreasing the infusion rate or using a weaker concentration of local anaesthetic.

Local anaesthetic drugs are capable of affecting sodium channels in all cells, not just nerve cells. Generally toxicity does not occur because the drug is injected close to the site of action and only diffuses slowly away into the circulatory system resulting in a low systemic concentration. However, if a large total mass of drug is injected toxicity can occur; this is related to the blocking of the sodium channels in the brain and heart.

Progressive side effects of local anaesthetic toxicity are:

- tinnitus, perioral numbness;
- restlessness;
- muscle twitching;
- loss of consciousness;
- generalised convulsions;
- respiratory arrest;
- hypotension;
- asystole (bupivacaine can produce ventricular arrhythmias).

Cardiovascular Adverse Effects of Local Anaesthetics

Vasodilatation of blood vessels can occur, causing relative hypovolaemia and tachycardia, with a resultant drop in blood pressure. This is exacerbated by blockade of the sympathetic nerve supply to the adrenal glands, preventing the release of catecholamines. If blockade is as high as T2, sympathetic supply to the heart (T2–T5) is also interrupted and may lead to bradycardia. The overall result may be inadequate perfusion of vital organs and measures are required to restore the blood pressure and cardiac output, such as fluid administration and the use of vasoconstrictors. Sympathetic outflow extends from T1 to L2 and blockade of nerve roots below this level (i.e. for lower limb surgery) is less likely to cause significant sympathetic blockade, compared with procedures requiring blockade above the umbilicus.

Respiratory Adverse Effects of Local Anaesthetics

The respiratory system is usually unaffected by local anaesthetic unless blockade is high enough to affect the intercostal muscle nerve supply (thoracic nerve roots) leading to reliance on diaphragmatic breathing alone and a reduced ability to cough or take a deep breath. This is likely to cause distress to the patient because he or she may feel unable to breathe adequately. If the block reaches upper cervical levels, bilateral phrenic nerve block may result in apnoea.

Visceral Adverse Effects of Local Anaesthetics

Urinary retention is a common problem with epidural analgesia. A severe drop in blood pressure may affect glomerular filtration in the kidney if sympathetic blockade extends high enough to cause significant vasodilatation. Urinary retention can also occur owing to sacral autonomic block.

Gastrointestinal Adverse Effects of Local Anaesthetics

Blockade of sympathetic outflow (T5–L1) to the gastrointestinal system leads to predominance of parasympathetic (vagus and sacral parasympathetic) outflow. This leads to active peristalsis, relaxed sphincters and a small contracted gut. Splenic enlargement (two- to threefold) can also occur.

Endocrine Adverse Effects of Local Anaesthetic

Nerve supply to the adrenals is blocked leading to a reduction in the release of catecholamines.

Local anaesthetic drugs are frequently used in combination with opioids in order to optimise the useful effects and minimise the undesirable effects of each drug. However, either of these classes of drugs can be used in isolation.

OPIOIDS

The analgesic and euphoric properties of opium have been known for hundreds of years. Opium is derived from the juice of unripe seed heads of the poppy (*Papaver somniferum*). The naturally occurring derivatives of opium are known as opiates and include morphine and diamorphine. Synthetic analogues of opium are known as opioids and include pethidine and fentanyl. Opioids is the term used to describe all these compounds which are the most useful drugs for treating acute pain, despite their associated side effects.

Direct application of opioids to the spinal cord through the epidural route provides excellent analgesia at much lower doses than are needed with systemic administration.

Pharmacodynamics of Opioids

Opioids mimic the action of the endogenous (naturally occurring) opioid peptides enkephalin, endorphin and dynorphin. Opioids provide pain relief by binding to opioid receptors in the spinal cord and brain. When injected into the epidural space a portion of the opioid binds to the epidural fat, a portion is absorbed into the epidural veins and a portion crosses the dura into the CSF. Once in the CSF a part of the dose is taken up by the spinal cord where it binds to the opioid receptors in the grey matter of the dorsal horn known as the substantia gelatinosa (Cox, 2002). The action of binding of opioids to the receptor sites decreases the release of the neurotransmitters that transmit painful impulses.

Pharmacokinetics of Opioids

The action of epidural opioids is influenced by their lipid solubility (the speed at which they will diffuse into fatty tissue). The degree of lipid solubility determines the rate of penetration of the drug through lipid membranes. The more lipid soluble the drug the quicker it will reach its site of action in the neural tissues. Morphine has low lipid solubility and so a slow onset of action, approximately 30 minutes after a bolus epidural injection. Pethidine and diamorphine have intermediate lipid solubility and will begin to exhibit an effect after approximately 15 minutes and fentanyl which has a high lipid solubility has a rapid onset of action of approximately 5 minutes (Cox, 2002).

Opioids are eliminated by diffusion into the bloodstream. Highly lipid soluble opioids are removed most rapidly from the epidural space and the CSF compared with those drugs with low lipid solubility. Therefore the effects of epidural fentanyl will last for a maximum of six hours compared with the long acting effects of morphine which have been described as being between 12 and 16 hours (Cox, 2002).

Adverse Effects of Opioids

Opioids, unlike local anaesthetics, do not have a direct effect on spinal nerves, so analgesia can be achieved without hypotension and sensory block or motor paralysis. However, there are a number of other significant adverse effects that are associated with opioid use regardless of the route of administration.

Respiratory Depression

Respiratory depression is a slowing of the respiratory rate and lower tidal volume; it is more likely to occur if the opioid used has low lipid solubility such as morphine than with highly lipid soluble drugs such as fentanyl. This is because morphine diffuses more slowly into the neural tissues, remaining in the CSF for prolonged periods, and is then transported in the CSF to the respiratory centre in the brain causing respiratory depression up to 24 hours after administration.

Patients receiving opioids via an epidural infusion should always have regular assessment of the level and character of respirations, sedation and oxygen saturations (Chapter 8). Less than eight breaths per minute is usually accepted as the indicator for respiratory depression (although the patient's baseline respiratory rate and sedation score must also be taken into consideration). The adverse effects of respiratory depression can be reversed using the specific opioid antagonist naloxone. Reliable venous access is essential so that naloxone may be administered intravenously if respiratory depression does occur.

Concurrent use of enteral or parenteral opioids should be avoided as this can significantly add to the risk of respiratory depression occurring.

Over-Sedation

Over-sedation may lead to respiratory depression owing to absorption of opioids into the circulation and delivery to the respiratory centre in the brain. The use of a sedation scoring tool is a useful way of measuring sedation or conscious level (Chapter 8). The epidural infusion should be stopped in patients who are somnolent or difficult to rouse.

Pruritus

Pruritus or itching is thought to result from the activation of opioid receptors in the spinal cord (Chapter 10) (Irvine and Wallace, 1997).

The incidence of pruritus varies, it is more common with morphine but can occur with all other opioids. The distribution is not related to the area of analgesia, but usually occurs around the head and neck area, although in some patients it is more generalised. It can be treated with low dose opioid antagonist naloxone, supporting the theory that it is an opioid receptor mediated central mechanism (Kyriakides *et al.*, 1999). It also responds to antihistamine drugs, e.g. chlorphenamine (Piriton) (Irvine and Wallace, 1997) and to the antiemetic serotonin antagonist ondansetron (Kyriakides *et al.*, 1999). It is sometimes possible to reduce the effects of pruritus by changing the opioid in the epidural infusion or removing the opioid and running a plain local anaesthetic epidural.

Nausea and Vomiting

The mechanism that supports opioid induced nausea and vomiting involves stimulation of serotonin and dopamine receptors in the chemoreceptor trigger zone (CTZ) of the brain by toxic substances. Neurotransmitters are then sent to the true vomit centre, which initiates the event of vomiting.

Some patients are deemed to be at high risk of nausea and vomiting, the risk factors are multifactorial including age, gender, obesity, history of postoperative nausea and vomiting (PONV), motion sickness, migraine, operative procedure being performed, anxiety, gastric stasis, certain anaesthetic agents and antibiotics (Cox, 1999). High risk patients should receive prophylactic antiemetic therapy and also a multimodal antiemetic approach may be beneficial.

Antiemetic drugs that work either directly or indirectly on the CTZ such as cyclizine, prochlorperazine, granisetron or ondansetron are the most likely to reduce the effects of opioid related nausea and vomiting.

Urinary Retention

Opioids in the CSF inhibit the volume induced bladder contractions and block the vesico-somatic reflex required for sphincter relaxation. Therefore, it may be possible to reverse the effects by the administration of low dose naloxone as it is thought to reverse the inhibition of sacral parasympathetic nervous system outflow that causes detrusor muscle relaxation leading to an increased maximal bladder capacity (Gravlee and Panick, 1993; Chaney, 1995). However, urinary retention associated with the epidural infusion is thought to be associated with the use of both opioid and local anaesthetic agents (Shafer and Donnelly, 1991), therefore naloxone may not be effective and urinary catheterisation may be required.

EPIDURAL PRESCRIPTIONS

Legal responsibility for prescribing lies with the anaesthetist (or other doctor) who signs the prescription. General guidance for good prescribing suggests that the medical practitioner should have taken time to explain to the patient the benefits and potential adverse effects of the medications to be prescribed. This should have formed part of the preoperative visit of the anaesthetist (Chapter 2).

When writing a prescription there are a number of important guidelines.

1. Prescriptions should be written legibly.
2. Indelible ink should be used.
3. Prescriptions should be dated.
4. The patient's full name, address and hospital number should appear on the prescription.
5. The name/number of the ward/department should appear on the prescription.
6. The doctor must sign the prescription (initials will not suffice).
7. Where possible the doctor's name and bleep number should be printed on the prescription.
8. Prescriptions for children should be completed with the child's age and/or date of birth.
9. Known allergies or sensitivities should appear on the hospital drug chart.
10. Drug names should be written in full and generic names should be used.
11. The route of administration should appear on the chart.
12. Grams should be written as g.
13. Fractions of grams should be written in mg.
14. Fractions of a milligram should be written in micrograms (mcg is not acceptable).
15. A zero should be included before the decimal point where decimals cannot be avoided.

Supplementary Prescribing

Supplementary prescribing has become a big part of the NHS modernisation agenda and there is growing evidence to suggest that nurse prescribing can have a considerable impact on improving the quality and appropriateness of care provided to patients (Hay *et al.*, 2004). Clinical nurse specialists are often more readily accessible to patients than anaesthetic colleagues, and therefore ideally placed to act as supplementary prescribers. They can provide a holistic package of care to meet some of the generic needs of patients who undergo major surgical procedures or sustain significant trauma. These needs include the provision of good pain relief and management of associated side effects such as respiratory depression, nausea and vomiting, pruritis and constipation.

Supplementary prescribing is a voluntary prescribing partnership between an independent prescriber, in this case the consultant anaesthetist, and a supplementary prescriber, the clinical nurse specialist (CNS). Both parties may visit the patient preoperatively and with the patient's agreement set up a clinical management plan (CMP) which can be utilised postoperatively (Figure 4.1).

The CMP must be patient specific and should include the patient's name, condition to be treated and relevant past medical history. The date, classes of

Patient Code No: Code number	Patient medication sensitivities/allergies:
Patient age / DOB:	

Past medical history	
Enter relevant past medical history	

Independent Prescriber(s):	Supplementary Prescriber(s)
Name	Name

Condition(s) to be treated	Aim of treatment
Postoperative pain	To reduce pain and increase quality of life

Medicines that may be prescribed by SP:

Preparation	Indication	Dose schedule	Specific indications for referral back to the IP
Paracetamol	Nociceptive pain	1g QDS	Medication is indicated which is not currently on the CMP
NSAIDs (diclofenac or ibuprofen)	Nociceptive pain	Dosing as per BNF	
Cyclizine			
	Nausea +/- vomiting	50 mg TDS	
Naloxone			
	Respiratory depression	Up to a maximum of 400 µg in incremental doses	
Epidural solution of fentanyl 4µg/ml and bupivacaine 0.125%	Nociceptive pain	Background rate between 2–8 ml per hour. Bolus dose of 2–5 ml and lock out time of 20 min.	
Weak opioid (Tramadol or co-codamol)	Nociceptive pain as a step-down preparation after discontinuation of epidural	Dosing as per BNF	
Oramorph	Nociceptive pain as a rescue during step-down preparation after discontinuation of epidural	5–10 mg 2 hourly PRN	

Guidelines or protocols supporting Clinical Management Plan:

WHO analgesic ladder
NICE guidelines for NSAIDs
Local protocol for naloxone
BNF

Frequency of review and monitoring by:

Supplementary prescriber 2 hourly monitoring by ward staff, twice daily review by CNS	Supplementary prescriber and independent prescriber Discussion with independent prescriber at once per week

Process for reporting ADRs:
Minor ADRs to be documented in patient's notes, medication reviewed.
Severe ADRs to be discussed with IP urgently and medication reviewed.
Unusual ADRs reported via Yellow card system by SP after discussion with IP.

Shared record to be used by IP and SP:
Medical notes

Agreed by independent prescriber(s)	Date	Agreed by supplementary prescriber(s)	Date	Date agreed with patient/carer

Figure 4.1. Clinical management plan.

medicines that may be prescribed, any restrictions or limitations and relevant warnings about patient sensitivities should be documented. Arrangements for notification of adverse drug reactions and the circumstances in which the supplementary prescriber should refer back to the independent prescriber must also be specified (Welsh Assembly Government, 2004).

Preprinted Labels

The RCA *et al.* (2004) suggest that safety is enhanced by the use of standard preprinted prescriptions for epidural infusion rather than relying on handwritten prescriptions that might be misinterpreted. Preprinted prescriptions may take the form of adhesive labels that can be stuck on to the patient's drug chart in an appropriate place. Labels should not be generally accessible; they should be stored in a limited number of places, i.e. anaesthetic rooms. They must also be individually signed and dated by the anaesthetist only at the time of use. Alternatively, preprinted dedicated monitoring charts that include the prescription can be used.

Dedicated Epidural Monitoring Charts with Incorporated Prescriptions

It is useful to devise and use dedicated epidural monitoring charts, which allow all of the relevant information to be held in one place. This type of chart can also incorporate all of the detail of the prescription for the epidural, provided there is reference to it on the patient's medication chart. The prescription should include the drugs and their concentrations, the rate in millilitres (ml) per hour to be infused (the rate should never be calculated in milligrams (mg) or micrograms (μg) per hour), and if a patient controlled epidural analgesia (PCEA) system is being utilised the size of the bolus dose in millilitres and also the lock out period in minutes.

It is also useful to incorporate a prescription for the opioid antagonist (where opioids are being utilised within the epidural solution) so that if prompt reversal is required in the case of severe respiratory depression the prescription is available.

Co-prescribing

No other opioid based analgesia (including codeine preparations) should be co-prescribed alongside the epidural if an opioid is contained within the epidural cocktail, as this will increase the risk of respiratory depression. There may be some exceptions with long-term opioid users, but careful discussion and the development of a treatment plan should be drawn up by the anaesthetist and CNS prior to insertion of the epidural catheter. Also closer monitoring of these patients is required for the duration of the epidural infusion.

There are other medications that should be co-prescribed including an opioid antagonist, oxygen, balanced analgesia and an appropriate antiemetic.

Naloxone

Naloxone, a synthetic opioid antagonist, should always be prescribed whenever an opioid is being administered. Naloxone competes with opioids for the opioid receptor sites in order to displace opioids and inhibit their action (McCaffery and Passero, 1999). Naloxone reverses not only the respiratory depressive effects of the opioid, but also the analgesic effects, therefore it is important to administer the drug in small titrated doses. The half-life of naloxone is shorter than the half-life of the opioid, so the effects will wear off while the opioid is still active putting the patient at further risk of respiratory depression.

Oxygen

Oxygen should also be prescribed to patients who receive epidural analgesia. It is given initially to patients after surgery on reversal of anaesthesia to encourage the transport of anaesthetic gases across the alveolar/capillary membrane in the lungs and out of the body. Supplementary oxygen is often required post-surgery because the metabolic changes that occur increase the body's oxygen requirements and if the patient is unable to meet the body's demand for increased oxygenation then respiratory failure can ensue (Clancy and McVicar, 2002). This potential respiratory problem coupled with the potential for opioid induced respiratory depression means that careful monitoring of oxygen saturation levels and respiratory activities is essential (Chapter 8).

Balanced Analgesia

Good quality analgesia cannot be achieved with single agents; it is much more likely to be achieved using a multimodal approach. Instead of relying on one class of drug to treat the pain a variety of drug groups, acting at different points in the pain pathway, is used. There is a wealth of evidence to suggest that smaller doses of each drug can be used and dose dependent side effects are reduced while analgesia is improved due to the synergistic effect gained (Stannard and Booth, 1998).

Step-Down Analgesia

Step-down analgesia should be put into place once a decision is made to discontinue the epidural. This should be done adhering to the World Health

Organisation analgesic ladder and stepping down from the top of the ladder (severe pain – strong opioid + NSAID + simple analgesic agent) to the middle of the ladder (moderate pain – weak opioid + NSAID + simple analgesic agent). First dosing of the step-down analgesic agents should occur approximately 30 minutes prior to the epidural being discontinued so that the oral analgesia begins to exert an effect when the epidural is stopped.

REFERENCES

Chaney, M. (1995) Side effects of intrathecal and epidural opioids. *Canadian Journal of Anesthesia*, **42** (10), 891–903.

Clancy, J. and McVicar, A. (2002) *Physiology and Anatomy: A Homeostatic Approach*, 2nd edn. London: Arnold.

Cox, F. (1999) Systematic review of ondansetron for the prevention and treatment of postoperative nausea and vomiting in adults. *British Journal of Theatre Nursing*, **9** (12), 556–66.

Cox, F. (2002) Making sense of epidural analgesia. *Nursing Times*, **98** (37), 56–8.

Gravlee, G. and Panick, R. (1993) *Pain Management in Cardio-Thoracic Surgery*. Philadelphia: Lippincott.

Hay, A., Bradley, A. and Nolan, P. (2004) Supplementary nurse prescribing. *Nursing Standard*, **18** (41), 33–42.

Irvine, G. and Wallace, M. (1997) *Pain Management for the Practicing Physician*. New York: Churchill.

Kyriakides, K., Hussain, S. and Hobbs, G. (1999) Management of opioid induced pruritus: a role for 5-Ht3 antagonists? *British Journal of Anaesthesia*, **82** (3), 439–41.

McCaffery, M. and Passero, C. (1999) *Pain Clinical Manual*, 2nd edn. St Louis: Mosby.

Melzack, R. and Wall, P. (1965) Pain mechanisms: a new theory. *Science*, **150**, 971.

Royal College of Anaesthetists and Pain Society (2003) *Pain Management Services – Good Practice*. London: RCA.

Royal College of Anaesthetists, Royal College of Nursing, the Association of Anaesthetists of Great Britain and Ireland, the British Pain Society and the European Society of Regional Anaesthesia and Pain Therapy (2004) *Good Practice in the Management of Continuous Epidural Analgesia in the Hospital Setting*. London: RCA.

Shafer, A. and Donnelly, A. (1991) Management of Postoperative Pain by Continuous Epidural Infusions of Analgesics. *Clinical Pharmacology*, **10** (11), 824.

Stannard, C. and Booth, S. (1998) *Churchill's Pocketbook of Pain*. Edinburgh: Churchill Livingstone.

Welsh Assembly Government (2004) *Supplementary Prescribing in Wales a Guide for Implementation*. Cardiff: WAG.

5

Epidural Delivery Systems

CAROLYN MIDDLETON[1] and LYNDA JENKINS[2]
[1]Clinical Nurse Specialist in Pain Management, Nevill Hall Hospital,
Abergavenny, South Wales
[2]Clinical Nurse Specialist in Pain Management, Morriston Hospital, Swansea,
South Wales

Dedicated equipment should be utilised to ensure safe and effective delivery of epidural solution to patients. This chapter aims to give healthcare professionals an overview of the specialised equipment required for epidural infusions and a review of the risk management issues relating to implementing a ward based service. Finally, the concept of patient controlled epidural analgesia (PCEA) delivery will be introduced.

DEDICATED EPIDURAL DEVICE

To ensure patient safety the equipment used to deliver epidural infusions should be exclusively designed for epidural use and should be configured accordingly. The device should also be standardised throughout the hospital or trust so that it becomes familiar to all staff involved in providing or supervising epidural infusions. Healthcare professionals that use epidural devices must be trained in their safe use (Chapter 4) and a manufacturer's pump specific handbook should be available to all users of the device (Royal College of Anaesthetists (RCA) et al., 2004).

The device should have specific built in safety features that allow:

Epidural Analgesia in Acute Pain Management. Edited by Carolyn Middleton.
© 2006 by John Wiley & Sons, Ltd. ISBN 0-470-01964-6

- programming to be delivered in millilitres per hour (rather than milligrams or micrograms per hour);
- rate capping so that the device can be configured with preset maximum infusion rate and bolus size;
- printable extended history available via key stroke logging to be used by the electrobiomedical engineering department (EBME) in the case of a clinical incident occurring;
- locking with restricted access to pain team and anaesthetic staff only;
- clear vision of fluids without unlocking the lockbox;
- adjustable pressure limits (limits determined by manufacturer);
- bolus administration by specialist users via lock facility (pain team and anaesthetic staff only);
- bolus administration by patients in the form of patient controlled epidural analgesia (PCEA).

Guidance and Legislation

There are clear guidance documents that steer the use and maintenance of medical devices, these including the 'MDA DB 9801 medical devices and equipment management for hospital and community based organisations', the 'MDA DB 9801 supplement one checks and tests for newly delivered medical devices' and the 'Welsh Risk Management Standard 30 medical equipment and devices'. There are also a number of legislative documents controlling the use of infusion devices. These include:

1. The Health and Safety at Work Act 1974
2. The Management of Health and Safety at Work Regulations 1992
3. The Provision and Use of Work Equipment Regulations 1998
4. The Electricity at Work Regulations 1989
5. The Electromagnetic Compatibility Directive 89/339/EEC 1989
6. The Workplace (Health, Safety and Welfare) Regulations 1992
7. The Medical Devices Directive 93/42/EEC June 1993.

There should be maintenance contracts in place either locally or with the manufacturer and all equipment must be subject to service test performance and verification procedures. Where work is undertaken locally, engineering departments (electrobiomedical engineering (EBME)) should follow work instructions based upon the manufacturer's guidance, which can be obtained from the manufacturer's operating and service instruction manuals. The frequency of service of devices can vary between manufacturers and device models, although it is recommended that devices are subject to one annual maintenance service which includes a full function and electrical safety test. All service and repair records must be retained on file using an equipment management database. There should also be in place a rolling replacement programme for equipment (RCA/Pain Society, 2003).

Labelling of Devices

All infusion devices should be labelled denoting the device performance type, risk category and an in-date electrical safety test. Each device should also carry an individual identification number; this number should be transcribed on to the patient's monitoring chart so that in the case of a clinical incident occurring the history information from the pump can be matched to other information gained from various monitoring charts pertaining to a named patient. Unlabelled epidural devices should not be used.

Dedicated Lines

Epidural infusion lines must be clearly identified; it would be advantageous to have a universally agreed standard colour for epidural infusion lines. In many hospitals yellow lines are used to signify epidural infusions (although there are various coloured lines available). Coloured products should however not be relied upon entirely for product identification; labelling should also be used. A preprinted label can be attached near to any connector at both ends of each line that clearly states the word 'epidural'. This type of labelling system makes the line easily recognisable when connecting the tubing. This system is used in an attempt to try to reduce the risk of an epidural line being connected to any other form of intravenous (IV) device or cannula.

The tubing utilised to connect the epidural device to the epidural catheter must be appropriate for the required flow rates (this information can usually be found in the manufacturer's handbook); many manufacturers have dedicated giving sets that are not universal. The giving sets which constitute the epidural system between the pump and the patient must be considered as a closed system and should not be breached, nor should they include injection ports (RCA *et al.*, 2004).

Antisiphon Valve

Where tubing (an epidural infusion line) is used to move a liquid from a higher location (an epidural pump) to a lower location (the patient), once the liquid starts to move down the pipe a vacuum develops at the lower location which sucks liquid from the upper location. This is known as a siphoning effect. This can cause an overdose of epidural solution being delivered and in the worst case scenario death can ensue. In order to prevent any siphoning effect from occurring and therefore protecting the patient, an antisiphon valve must be fitted. This usually takes the form of a small valve fitted on to the epidural line nearest to the connector with the pump. Some lines have a built in antisiphon feature, and others require the valve to be attached separately.

The pump should also be located at a height that is approximately the same as the patient's chest height. If the pump is too high or too low again the siphoning effect is more likely to occur.

Antibacterial Filter

An antibacterial filter must always be used in the infusion line at the junction between the epidural catheter and the infusion line. This filter is used in an attempt to minimise the risk of intraluminar bacterial contamination by excluding bacteria and microscopic debris from the epidural and preventing potential development of an epidural abscess (Chapter 10). The filter should be transparent to allow visual monitoring of filtration. Care should be taken to ensure that the filter does not cause a pressure sore and for this reason many filters are manufactured in the shape of a flat disc specifically to enhance patient comfort (Figure 5.1). Regardless of the profile there should be regular assessment of the skin under the filter. Some filters are designed with a self-adhesive fixative system to keep the filter in place (as shown in Figure 5.1).

There is little good quality evidence to guide practice regarding the changing of the antibacterial filter or epidural administration set, therefore practice should be directed by the manufacturer's instructions and local policy. It is generally accepted that filters should not be changed as this can increase the risk of contamination.

Device Alarm Systems

All epidural devices should have alarm systems which are designed to notify the healthcare professional of any potential problems. It should be noted that patients sometimes worry when hearing a device alarm for the first time; reassurance is required from the nurse and it may be useful to provide the patients with an explanation of the alarm system at the preoperative visit.

Examples of device alarms are: an occlusion in the line, a severely depleted reservoir of epidural or air in the giving set. International standards require that infusion devices have a system in place that is sophisticated enough to detect single bubbles of 1.1 ml of air and trigger an alarm system. Every effort should be made to eradicate air from the system although a small amount of air in the epidural space is not likely to cause problems (air can be used to test for loss of resistance when inserting the epidural catheter – see Chapter 3).

Specific actions for responding to alarm calls should be set out in the local policy and should also be included in the competency based training (Chapter 11).

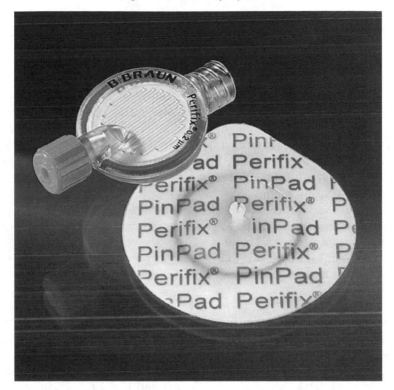

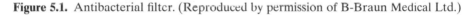

Figure 5.1. Antibacterial filter. (Reproduced by permission of B-Braun Medical Ltd.)

RESUSCITATION

In every ward or department area where epidural infusions are used there should always be access to appropriate resuscitation equipment and drugs. The RCA *et al.* (2004) state that there must be 24 hour availability of staff competent to recognise and manage the more serious complications including cardiorespiratory resuscitation.

PATIENT LOCATION

Where a patient is managed following surgery with an epidural in progress may vary. A study reviewing epidural practice of 214 training hospitals in the UK found that just over half of the departments (54%) managed their patients on the wards. The other 46% were managed exclusively in the intensive care or high dependency unit (Cook *et al.*, 1997). Those hospitals that rarely used epidural analgesia restricted the practice to high dependency care areas which can severely restrict the numbers of epidurals that are performed.

Patients should only be cared for in general surgical wards if the hospital can provide:

- easily visible areas for constant surveillance and nursing support;
- nursing education programmes to ensure all staff are competent to safely manage patients receiving epidural infusion;
- continuous 24 hour monitoring and documentation of pain scores, respiratory rate, conscious level, height of block, assessment of motor function, monitoring of blood pressure, urine output and inspection of epidural site;
- nurses available who are trained to change infusion rates and/or solutions and are familiar with the infusion pumps used;
- designated infusion pumps;
- an acute pain service which is available to provide: protocols, policies and/or guidelines, common solutions to problems, daily review of patients receiving epidural infusions and regular audit of the service;
- good communication must exist between ward nurses, pain team and anaesthetic staff to ensure coordinated management.

(RCA *et al.*, 2004)

Numerous studies have shown that epidural analgesia can provide better analgesia and fewer complications than intravenous opioid infusions on general surgical wards providing there is vigilance and a robust supporting structure is in place for both patients and staff (Ready *et al.*, 1991; Hobbs and Roberts *et al.*, 1992; Leith *et al.*, 1994; Schug and Fry, 1994; Rygnestad *et al.*, 1997; Liu *et al.*, 1998).

RISK MANAGEMENT

All activities carry risks and using epidural devices is no exception. Faults can occur with any piece of equipment, therefore epidural devices should be checked before use and after accidental damage such as dropping. Equipment that is thought to be faulty should never be used; the fault must be reported to the EBME department.

In order to reduce the risks associated with epidural infusion there should be an appropriate training programme for staff in place (Chapter 11). A risk management exercise should have been undertaken identifying the possible risks associated with epidural infusion. For each possible risk a calculation should be performed of how likely it is to occur and the severity of potential outcomes. Where necessary, strategies need to be implemented to reduce the identified risks. A policy should be in place for the safe use of epidural devices along with an appropriate reporting system if incidents do occur.

CLINICAL INCIDENTS

If an error, clinical incident or near miss occurs, practitioners must ensure that the trust/hospital clinical incident reporting procedure is implemented. Many trusts operate a 'no blame' culture and actively encourage incident reporting in order to:

- improve patient care;
- prevent reoccurrences of incidents;
- identify trends;
- review existing practices;
- identify additional training needs;
- respond to complaints.

If a clinical incident does occur the immediate priority is the clinical management of the patient. An adverse clinical incident form should be completed and the pain team or anaesthetist should be informed along with relevant nurses and risk managers. The epidural device must be immediately removed from clinical use. On removal all readings and settings must be recorded and left unchanged. All elements of the device and giving set must be left intact and clearly labelled with a declaration of contamination status. The nurse in charge of the area must then forward the device to the EBME department as soon as possible.

Pain services should have in place an integrated system covering management, reporting, analysis and learning from adverse incidents (DoH, 2001).

Epidural Solution

In each hospital there should be a strict limitation on the number and concentration of drugs used for epidural infusions. The prescription outlining the drugs and concentrations should be clearly described in local protocols and/or guidelines; any variation from these protocols should occur only in exceptional circumstances and be ratified where possible by the consultant anaesthetist with responsibility for the pain service.

For safety, preprepared solutions should be utilised. These solutions should be prepared aseptically in a special unit either by a local appropriately equipped pharmacy department or by an outside manufacturer and then bought in. This reduces the risk of drug error in the preparation of the solution and it reduces the possibility of introducing bacteria into the epidural bag or syringe.

Clear labelling must be used to distinguish epidural infusion solutions from all other infusion solutions used within the hospital. Epidural solutions should be stored separately from solutions intended for intravenous usage; dedicated epidural controlled drugs cupboards (where opioids are used within the cocktail) are preferable. Yellow labels are often used to label epidural bags or syringes in the UK; yellow is the colour that has been adopted to signify epidurals (although the clinician should never rely on colour coding alone and should read and check the drug label carefully).

EPIDURAL MODE OF DELIVERY

Traditionally epidural infusions were delivered via continuous infusion only. If the rate of infusion was not sufficient to provide analgesia it required review followed by pump manipulation to increase the delivery rate or to administer a clinician bolus in an attempt to make the patient more comfortable. Extensive experience has been gained with intravenous patient controlled analgesia (PCA) devices, which has been used to inform epidural modes of delivery. Patient controlled systems have been shown to improve patient satisfaction and decrease labour workload of the staff. Patient controlled epidural analgesia (PCEA) provides an exciting development in epidural practice.

PCEA

PCEA was introduced because it was predicted that it would offer several potential advantages over continuous infusion or bolus only administration methods. These include increased patient autonomy, easy titration of sensory level, high patient satisfaction and a reduced demand on professional time. However, in many hospitals patient delivery systems are still a relatively new concept and at an early stage of development.

The use of the continuous epidural infusion plus a demand dose mode has been described by Ferrante *et al.* (1991) as a 'hybrid' of patient and physician controlled analgesia. The PCEA system of delivery eradicates changing of rates and intermittent clinician top-up boluses (Liu *et al.*, 1998). There have been several clinical trials that have directly compared the efficacy of PCEA with a continuous only epidural system. In all cases PCEA has been shown to be as effective, and in most cases analgesic efficacy of the PCEA system has proved to be superior to continuous only delivery system (Boudreault *et al.*, 1991). There have also been reported psychological benefits when patients are able to control their own pain management.

By adding a patient controlled bolus system it is possible that the iatrogenic over-administration of epidural solution from a continuous infusion system may be prevented. Lower continuous background rates can be utilised if the patient has the ability to increase the epidural dose in relation to pain experience. Therefore, there may be fewer adverse events with PCEA than with a continuous only delivery.

Close monitoring of respiratory rate is essential in patients receiving epidural analgesia via both continuous only and PCEA with or without a background infusion because absorption of opioids into the circulatory system and subsequent delivery to the respiratory centre in the brain stem can result in respiratory depression.

Infusion Rates

The infusion rate and bolus dose size should be influenced by the patient's age and general condition. There is an age related decrease in the volume of local anaesthetic needed to achieve a given level of block. This is because there is likely to be a greater spread from a single dose of local anaesthetic in elderly patients owing to a decrease in the size and compliance of the epidural space.

The patient's height also appears to correlate to some extent with the volume of local anaesthetic needed to produce an analgesic effect. An adult of 1.5 m should therefore have lower infusion rates prescribed than taller patients. There is little correlation between the weight of a patient and the volume of local anaesthetic needed, although in morbidly obese patients the epidural space may be compressed because of increased intra-abdominal pressure, and a smaller volume of local anaesthetic is therefore needed.

The combination of an opioid with a local anaesthetic (epidural cocktail) is thought to allow lower rates of infusion than using either drug in isolation. Also, lower infusion rates can be used with higher concentrations of the epidural drugs. It must be remembered that increased concentrations will give more dense blocks rather than increased dermatomal spread.

The volume injected will influence the spread of the local anaesthetic following bolus administration. The greater the volume the greater the spread of the solution and therefore the greater the dermatomal area affected. This concept also applies to background rates; lower rates of infusion can be used if the level of epidural catheter insertion corresponds accurately to the level of dermatomal cover required. The level of insertion will also affect the spread of the infused solution, as there tends to be a greater spread in thoracic epidurals where the epidural space is smaller than in the lumbar area.

The position of the patient has traditionally been assumed to have a gravitational effect on the spread of local anaesthetic and therefore the area blocked. A patient in a sitting position will experience blockade of the lower lumbar and sacral roots. A patient in the lateral position will notice that the nerve roots on the dependent side are more densely blocked, although some anaesthetists have discounted this theory.

After lumbar injection, analgesia spreads both caudally and cranially, with a delay at the L5 and S1 segments, due to the large size of these nerve roots. When PCEA is being used, the total potential background and bolus dose per hour must be taken into consideration. The bolus dose should be such that sudden drops in blood pressure are unlikely, i.e. a bolus of 2–6 ml. The lockout time should be set to allow absorption of one bolus before the next bolus is accessible by the patient, therefore the recommended bolus should be between 15 and 25 minutes dependent on the lipid solubility of the drugs used (Chapter 4).

The force of the injection also has a notable effect, the greater the force of the injection, the greater the spread of the local anaesthetic. Delivery device infusion and bolus delivery rates are also regulated by the manufacturer's specification (details of which can be found in the device handbook).

DOCUMENTATION

Information relating to the epidural analgesia therapy, together with any complications, should be documented in the patient's record (Stannard and Booth, 1998). The anaesthetists, clinical nurse specialists (CNSs) and ward nursing staff all have a legal and professional responsibility to ensure good record keeping which will help to protect the welfare of patients by promoting:

- high standards of clinical care;
- continuity of care;
- better communication and dissemination of information between members of the multiprofessional healthcare team;
- an accurate account of treatment and care planning and delivery;
- the ability to detect problems such as changes in the patient's condition at an early stage (Nursing and Midwifery Council (NMC), 2005).

The quality of the records kept reflects the standard of professional practice; good records are the sign of a skilled and safe practitioner. The CNS should keep pain service records for each patient to allow tracking of caseload, they should also make appropriate entries into the multidisciplinary case notes held on the ward or department where the patient is being cared for. The documentation should be legible, factual, consistent and accurate. Records should be written at the time of reviewing the patient or as soon afterwards as possible. Each entry must be signed, dated and timed. Writing should be clear and free of any alterations. Deletions or additions should also be signed with the date and time entered. Abbreviations, jargon, speculation and offensive subjective statements should be avoided (NMC, 2005). Good record keeping is a tool of professional practice and not separate from the clinical care process – it is not an optional extra.

Information technology (IT) is being increasingly used within health care as a method of storing patient data. This system has the advantages that records are easier to read and less bulky; IT helps to reduce duplication and increase access and communication across the interprofessional healthcare team. CNSs are professionally accountable for making sure that the system used is robust and secure; the basic principle for computerised records is guided by the data protection legislation.

The period for which dedicated pain service patient records should be kept will depend on legislation and health service policy statements issued by the Department of Health. Local protocols will provide specific information, but generally records should be kept for at least eight years for adults and in the case of children at least until the date of their 21st birthday (NMC, 2005).

CODES OF PRACTICE

There are several codes of practice that relate to healthcare professionals that are relevant to the use of infusion devices, these include the 'Guidelines for the administration of medicines' (NMC, 2002), 'Guidelines for records and record keeping' (NMC, 2005 – as mentioned above), 'Medicines and healthcare products regulatory agency (MHRA) guidance on the use of infusion devices', the 'Welsh risk management standards' (Wales only) and the Nursing and Midwifery Council's 'Code of Professional Conduct' (NMC, 2002).

REFERENCES

Boudreault, D., Brasseur, L., Samii, K. and Lemoing, J. (1991) Comparison of continuous epidural bupivacaine infusion plus either continuous epidural infusion or patient controlled epidural injection of fentanyl for postoperative analgesia. *Anesthesia & Analgesia*, **73**, 132–7.

Cook, T., Eaton, J. and Goodwin, A. (1997) Epidural analgesia following upper abdominal surgery: United Kingdom practice. *Acta Anaesthesiology Scandinavia*, **41**, 18–24.

DoH (2001) Guidelines for preventing infections associated with the insertion and maintenance of central venous catheters. *Journal of Hospital Infection*, **47** (suppl), S47–S67.

Ferrante, F., Lu, L., Jamison, S. and Datta, S. (1991) Patient controlled epidural analgesia: demand dosing. *Anaesthesia & Analgesia*, **73** (5), 547–52.

Hobbs, G. and Roberts, F. (1992) Epidural infusion of bupivacaine and diamorphine for postoperative analgesia – use on general surgical wards. *Anaesthesia*, **47**, 58–62.

Leith, S., Wheatley, R., Jackson, L. and Hunter, D. (1994) Extra-dural infusion analgesia for postoperative pain relief. *British Journal of Anaesthesia*, **73**, 552–8.

Liu, S., Allen, H. and Olsson, G. (1998) Patient-controlled epidural analgesia with bupivacaine and fentanyl on hospital wards: prospective experience with 1,030 surgical patients. *Anaesthesiology*, **88**, 688–95.

Nursing and Midwifery Council (2002) *Guidelines for the Administration of Medicines*. London: NMC.

Nursing and Midwifery Council (2005) *Guidelines for Records and Record Keeping*. London: NMC.

Ready, L., Loper, K., Neesly, M. and Wild, L. (1991) Postoperative epidural morphine is safe on surgical wards. *Anaesthesiology*, **75**, 452–6.

Royal College of Anaesthetists and the Pain Society (2003) *Pain Management Services – Good Practice*. London: RCA.

Royal College of Anaesthetists, Royal College of Nursing, the Association of Anaesthetists of Great Britain and Ireland, the British Pain Society and the European Society of Regional Anaesthesia and Pain Therapy (2004) *Good Practice in the Management of Continuous Epidural Analgesia in the Hospital Setting*. London: RCA.

Rygnestad, T., Borchgrevink, P. and Eide, E. (1997) Postoperative epidural infusion of morphine and bupivacaine is safe on surgical wards. Organisation of the treatment, effects and side-effects in 2000 consecutive patients. *Acta Anaesthesiology Scandinavia*, **41**, 868–76.

Schug, S. and Fry, R. (1994) Continuous regional analgesia in comparison with intravenous opioid administration for routine postoperative pain control. *Anaesthesia*, **49**, 528–32.

Stannard, C. and Booth, S. (1998) *Churchill's Pocketbook of Pain*. Edinburgh: Churchill Livingstone.

6

Epidurals in Obstetrics

CAROLYN MIDDLETON

Clinical Nurse Specialist in Pain Management, Nevill Hall Hospital,
Abergavenny, South Wales

The painful experience of labour is as old as the human race itself (Steer, 1993). Obstetric epidural analgesia is used to provide relief from pain associated with labour and delivery by the administration of a local anaesthetic +/– an opioid into the epidural space. Epidural analgesia in childbirth has been the subject of much research over the past forty years and there is accumulating evidence to support its efficacy and safety compared with alternatives. Today epidural analgesia is considered to be the cornerstone of obstetric analgesic practice.

This chapter aims to provide an overview of obstetric pain mechanisms and pathways, along with specific issues relating to epidural analgesia during labour and delivery. Appropriate drugs, doses and delivery systems (which are constantly under review) are essential components of an obstetric epidural service; these issues will also be explored.

PAIN IN LABOUR

The intensity of pain in labour varies considerably although according to Russell et al. (1997) it is rated by the majority of women as being severe. Unlike other pains, labour pains are not associated with a pathological condition but with a physiological process. In the first stage of labour the

Epidural Analgesia in Acute Pain Management. Edited by Carolyn Middleton.
© 2006 by John Wiley & Sons, Ltd. ISBN 0-470-01964-6

pain increases in severity and frequency in line with uterine contractions. Uterine contraction pain is transmitted via visceral afferent fibres to the sympathetic chain and on to the first lumbar and the eleventh and twelfth thoracic segments of the spinal cord. This produces pain in both the abdomen and the back and the back pain may be exacerbated if the fetal head presses on the lumbosacral plexus.

In the second stage of labour, the pain maintains the features of the first stage but increases in severity owing to perineal distension as the baby's head descends through the birth canal. This pain is transmitted via the pudendal nerves to the second, third and fourth sacral segments of the spinal cord.

ALTERED PHYSIOLOGY IN PREGNANCY

There is normally a negative pressure in the epidural space; this is predominantly because of transmission of negative intrathoracic pressure through the intervertebral foramina. This negative pressure is greatest in the upper and middle thoracic regions and least in the lumbar and sacral regions. In the late stages of pregnancy, and the second stage of labour, this pressure increases to the point where a negative pressure in the epidural space can no longer be demonstrated. Pressure changes of this type within the body's cavities are reflected in the epidural veins, this is particularly notable in pregnancy when the veins become distended and engorged. This distension of the veins reduces the effective volume of the epidural space and increases the pressure within it. This effect can be extenuated when the expectant mother is in the sitting position.

In non-pregnant patients it is very rare for an epidural block to extend very high, but in pregnancy the risk is increased. Venous distension and the effects of progesterone reduce the compliance of the epidural space and in turn enhance the spread of epidural solution. Resuscitation equipment should therefore be readily available when epidural catheters are being placed in labouring women, although the block does usually recede quite quickly and monitoring and reassurance are all that are usually needed.

Aortocaval compression or occlusion occurs in all women at term, but some will display 'supine hypotensive syndrome of pregnancy'. The uterus compresses the vena cava and aorta against the lumbar spine causing a reduction in venous return to the heart and a reduction in uterine blood flow. Hypotension will ensue, compromising both mother and baby unless the patient is positioned laterally to maintain adequate circulation. Fluid resuscitation may be required, preloading of crystalloid solution is common as a preventive measure but it is controversial as it can be hazardous in patients with cardiac disease and reduced left ventricular compliance. If severe hypotension does occur, vasopressors such as ephedrine can be given.

CONSENT

The general principles of consent are described in Chapter 2 (local guidelines regarding obtaining consent need to be applied). Surveys suggest that in most cases anaesthetists do not obtain written consent for regional analgesia for labour pains. Obtaining consent for epidural insertion in a distressed labouring patient, who may be affected by drugs, is difficult and may not be informed; therefore it would not be legally valid. However, the anaesthetist is unlikely to face problems within the legal system provided discussion occurred and the patient was cooperative.

An example of an ethical dilemma that an anaesthetist may be presented with is when a patient writes a birth plan as an advanced directive stating that she does not, under any circumstances, even if she asks for it, want an epidural. Then during labour she becomes very distressed with pain and makes repeated requests for an epidural. Should she be told that she must stick to her birth plan and be denied this type of pain relief? Or should it be considered that she has the right to change her mind and make a new decision during labour, and be given an epidural? A decision has to be made regarding the patient's competency at the time of request and ultimately the anaesthetist makes the final decision based on the patient's best interests.

Expectant mothers cannot know in advance how painful their labour will be; neither can the midwife or anaesthetist predict this information. Scott (1991) suggests that a patient can only make an informed choice when she actually experiences the degree of pain involved. So when developing a birth plan these issues should be taken into consideration; a flexible approach is useful.

It is preferable that written and verbal information is given at an antenatal appointment when labour pains are not interfering with decision-making processes, consent can then be reaffirmed during labour. In all cases discussion should take place that includes an explanation of the procedure, evidence for efficacy, level of risk and individual patient expectations. The Royal College of Anaesthetists (RCA) (2001) has produced a booklet for patients outlining the advantages and disadvantages of epidurals (and other forms of pain relief) in labour this can be found on the Royal College of Anaesthetists' website at www.rcoa.ac.uk.

There is an expectation from mothers that epidural analgesia will provide excellent pain relief. Although the vast majority of epidurals do achieve this, complete relief from pain cannot be guaranteed. Ideally, obstetric units should be able to provide an epidural service on request at all times, but some units will only be able to provide an occasional service when appropriately trained anaesthetic staff are available. At booking women should be informed of the service they can expect so that expectations are realistic (Association of

Anaesthetists of Great Britain and Ireland (AAGBI) and Obstetric Anaesthetists Association, 1998).

POSSIBLE INDICATIONS FOR EPIDURAL ANALGESIA

Epidural analgesia can provide gold standard pain relief for women suffering labour related distress, those who have had a previous caesarean section and are undergoing trial of labour, women who have had an induced labour and those unfortunate women who have suffered an interuterine death.

There are also certain complications or conditions in pregnancy where an epidural is recommended for medical reasons.

- **Breech presentation**. Although many breech babies are delivered via caesarean section, some are delivered vaginally. Where there is an uncontrollable urge to push before the cervix is fully dilated oedema and bruising of the cervix ensues hampering delivery and causing significant risk to the baby. Epidural analgesia prevents uncontrolled pushing making a breech vaginal delivery safer.
- **Multiple births**. After the birth of the first baby in a multiple pregnancy uterine inertia, cord compression or partial separation of the placenta can occur which requires intervention. An effective epidural will allow an assisted delivery or caesarean section without the need to proceed to general anaesthesia. It may also reduce the time between delivery of the babies.
- **Occipito-posterior position**. Owing to the laxity of the pelvic floor, rotation of the fetal head may be delayed and may ultimately have to be performed manually or instrumentally. The long distressing labour of a primigravida with occipito-posterior presentation may be helped with an epidural (Beavis, 1984).
- **Pre-eclampsia/toxaemia**. Epidural analgesia in labour helps to rescue plasma catecholamine levels and reduce peripheral vascular resistance reducing blood pressure fluctuations associated with pain and contractions.
- **Premature labour**. Epidural analgesia avoids the effects of systemic opioids on the premature baby, it reduces premature pushing reflexes, prevents delivery through an undilated cervix and creates good conditions for intrauterine manipulation and controlled delivery.
- **Maternal morbidity**. There is increasing evidence to show that epidurals reduce or reverse the stress related responses of the body to pain and childbirth. There is a reduction in hyperventilation, increased muscle relaxation, reduction in blood pressure and an improvement in blood chemistry. The workload of the heart and the body's oxygen requirement are reduced and blood flow to the uterus is improved. So epidural analgesia benefits women

with severe asthma and other chronic respiratory conditions. Also the respiratory effects of systemic opioids are avoided and the ability to clear secretions is enhanced. In diabetic women epidurals reduce catecholamine and 11-hydroxycorticosteroid levels resulting in better maternal glucose control and placental profusion.

- **Maternal obesity**. A reduction of cardiopulmonary stress and better oxygenation in labour is achieved with epidural analgesia.

EPIDURAL CATHETER INSERTION

The anaesthetist should perform a risk–benefit analysis (for further information see Chapter 2). Epidurals like many other medical interventions have a list of potential problems associated with them; some are common but not serious, others are extremely rare but very serious such as permanent paralysis, cardiac arrest and death which occur in between 1 in 20000 and 1 in 1000000 patients in labour (RCA *et al.*, 2004).

There is also considerable benefit associated with epidural analgesia and it is the anaesthetist's role to ensure that the benefits outweigh the risks. In large hospitals it is common for approximately 50% of women to receive epidural analgesia in labour and around 90% for caesarean sections with a very good safety record which is largely due to the high standard of training of the anaesthetists (RCA and AAGBI, 2004).

For labour, epidurals are usually inserted between the second and fourth lumbar vertebrae. The epidural catheter should ideally be placed before the mother becomes greatly distressed; this makes the task of catheter insertion easier for the anaesthetist if the mother is co-operative and able to adequately flex her spine. Positioning can be difficult late in pregnancy making it technically harder to place the needle and subsequently the catheter into the epidural space.

MONITORING

It is imperative that safety standards are maintained to a level that ensures that serious complications associated with epidural analgesia are recognised early and appropriate remedial action taken. A trained midwife should provide continuous care and monitoring of the mother and fetus for the duration of the epidural infusion. The mother should be closely monitored and not left unattended for more than 20 minutes after each top-up of epidural solution. Women should be encouraged to report any adverse drug reactions to the attending nurse and/or medical staff (AAGBI and Obstetric Anaesthetists Association, 1998). The anaesthetic department has responsibility for units which offer a 24 hour on demand epidural analgesia service for women in labour and should therefore ensure the availability of an anaesthetist in the hospital at all times (AAGBI and Obstetric Anaesthetists Association, 1998).

Patient and pump observations set out in Chapter 8 should be regularly recorded and documented. These should include respiratory rate, sedation and pain scoring; recording of temperature, pulse and blood pressure; checking of the epidural catheter insertion site for any signs of infection and checking of the pump to ensure that the correct drugs are being delivered to the correct patient in the correct doses. Urinary output should also be recorded and bladder distension prevented. Finally, hourly assessment of the sensory and motor block should be recorded during the labour in a bid to ensure there is no significant degree of motor block present so that safe ambulation can take place (AAGBI and Obstetric Anaesthetists Association, 1998).

The baby's heart rate should be recorded before, during and after the establishment of the epidural infusion (AAGBI and Obstetric Anaesthetists Association, 1998).

EPIDURAL ANALGESIA FOR THE FIRST STAGE OF LABOUR

Epidural analgesia can provide effective pain relief during the typically long first stage of labour without causing excessive maternal sedation or mental confusion. The catheter is positioned in the epidural space between the second and fourth lumbar vertebrae near the nerves associated with the first stage of labour, the first lumbar and the eleventh and twelfth thoracic segments of the spinal cord. The local anaesthetic from the epidural is delivered in close proximity to these nerves producing very effective analgesia.

Epidurals can also provide excellent delivery conditions which can be particularly useful for complicated deliveries or where surgical intervention is anticipated (Paech, 2000).

MOBILE EPIDURAL

Motor block is a well documented consequence of epidural analgesia and precludes ambulation. The density of the block depends on local anaesthetic concentration, dose and duration of administration, therefore appropriate selection of epidural solution is essential if lower limb and abdominal muscle weakness is to be minimised. It is essential to have guidelines in place to test for motor power in the lower limbs prior to ambulation if patient falls are to be prevented.

Modern epidurals using low dose local anaesthetics reduce the risk of motor block and therefore allow adequate and safe mobility. Lower concentrations of local anaesthetic can be particularly effective when combined with opioids producing a synergistic effect (Paech, 2000). Increased mobility combined with good quality analgesia improves maternal satisfaction and increases patient autonomy (Collis *et al.*, 1995).

EPIDURAL ANALGESIA FOR THE SECOND STAGE OF LABOUR

The second stage of labour (delivery) begins at the time when the cervix has reached full dilation (10 cm) and the head has descended within the pelvis. At this point involuntary activity of the pelvic floor muscles occurs in synchrony with uterine contractions in order for the fetal head to be pushed through the open cervix and birth canal. The fetal head must then negotiate the changing diameter of the birth canal as it descends through it by assuming a series of changes in head position. These manoeuvres may fail to occur or may occur more slowly if the uterine or pelvic floor muscles are not contracting well. Voluntary contracting of the abdominal wall and pelvic muscles by the mother at this point will contribute to the effectiveness of the delivery.

Epidural analgesia is not usually associated with changes in the number of uterine contractions, but it may reduce pelvic floor tone and lower abdominal muscle power adversely affecting the voluntary maternal expulsive effort (Paech, 2000). The degree of effect will depend on the amount of motor block produced by the epidural. With full sensory loss the bearing down reflex will be missing which may increase the interval between full dilatation of the cervix and delivery.

In some hospitals there has been a deliberate attempt by the midwife, obstetrician or anaesthetist to restore a degree of sensation to the birth canal so that the mother is better able to coordinate her pushing with the bearing down reflex. To achieve this practice has been to withhold the epidural during the second stage of labour in order to reduce the possibility of extending delivery time. It has been argued that this practice does not reduce the rate of spontaneous delivery, but merely significantly increases the severity of maternal pain. This has been a controversial issue with considerable debate within the literature. Do epidurals actually increase the duration of labour? Meta-analyses have reported that epidural analgesia results in a slight increase in labour duration of 45 minutes in the first stage and 15 minutes in the second stage (Clarke *et al.*, 1998: Gambling *et al.*, 1990; Halpern *et al.*, 1998). However, there is no evidence that this delay is associated with any risks to the baby in a properly managed labour.

Epidurals may prove to be less effective in managing the second stage of labour pain regardless of any reduction in the amount of epidural solution being administered (although some degree of benefit will still be gained). Pain is transmitted in the second stage via the pudendal nerves to the second, third and fourth sacral segments of the spinal cord, this is not usually in close proximity to the epidural catheter insertion level and therefore the epidural solution has some distance to travel to reach these sacral nerves. This makes it less likely that the associated dermatomal areas will be adequately blocked unless there is an increase in volume of epidural solution injected. Therefore the epidural will be rendered less effective during the second stage of labour than it was during the first.

EPIDURALS AND THE INCIDENCE OF INSTRUMENTAL VAGINAL DELIVERY AND CAESAREAN SECTION RATES

Reports have suggested that high concentrations of local anaesthetic given as part of the epidural infusion can produce a dense motor blockade that alters the characteristics of the second stage of labour. Reduction in pelvic tone and lower abdominal muscle power can potentially affect the maternal expulsive efforts increasing the time between full dilation of the cervix and delivery. This can potentially increase the risk of instrumental delivery, particularly in first pregnancies (Halpern *et al.*, 1998).

Howell's (2004) systematic review of 11 randomised controlled trials (RCTs) (n = 3157) comparing epidural analgesia with other forms of analgesia (not involving regional blockade) concluded that epidural analgesia was associated with longer first and second stages of labour and instrumental vaginal delivery but there was no acceptable evidence that associates epidurals with an increased incidence of caesarean section rates (Howell, 2004). Therefore, the use of minimum effective doses of local anaesthetic should optimise safety and reduce such risks. A useful way of achieving this is to use a patient controlled epidural analgesia (PCEA) system which allows the mother to self-administer analgesia. There is much debate regarding which system of delivery of epidural solution is the more effective: continuous only delivery or PCEA with or without a background infusion.

Continuous infusions are thought to provide more uniform pain relief, but have the potential for an increased staff workload where intermittent bolus top-ups are required. PCEA has been shown to provide excellent pain relief, flexibility and patient autonomy maximising the mother's feelings of control during labour in determining her level of pain relief. It allows greater ability to titrate sensory level by reducing the amount of local anaesthetic required by 20–50% compared with background continuous infusion method, provided the bolus doses of dilute local anaesthetic are small and the lockout period is at least 15 minutes (Paech, 2000). Many women simply want their contractions to be made more tolerable; they do not want sensation abolished altogether. For these reasons many obstetric units now use PCEA systems for managing labour pains.

There is also the scenario that the need for an assisted instrumental delivery may have arisen as a result of factors unrelated to the epidural, which is often the case. Prolonged labours can be associated with fetal distress and maternal exhaustion, when this occurs it is sometimes necessary to speed up the delivery of the baby with the use of forceps or vacuum suction. In this event good pain relief may be required in the lower birth canal and perineum area. Higher concentrations of local anaesthetic may be required for this procedure to be carried out.

EPIDURAL DRUGS IN OBSTETRICS

For many years epidural local anaesthetics (LA) were used during labour in the same doses as were used for surgery, this proved to be effective in blocking pain transmission but was associated with numerous adverse events. However, when managed properly epidural analgesia has proved to be remarkably safe and the related side effects and serious complications tend to be rare and largely preventable.

The use of minimum effective doses of LA should optimise safety and reduce the risk of toxicity. Bupivacaine has a long duration of action and minimal plasma accumulation with repeat dosing, it is therefore usually the drug of choice (Paech, 2000). Newer drugs such as ropivacaine and levobupivacaine appear promising, their pharmacological properties are similar to bupivacaine but with less potential for toxicity. For further information regarding drugs and delivery systems see Chapter 4.

There is a plethora of evidence to demonstrate that the addition of opioids to epidural solutions allows a reduction in local anaesthetic dose and consequently a reduction in the incidence and severity of local anaesthetic side effects without compromising analgesia (Brownridge, 1991; Breen, 1996). This combination has a synergistic effect and is reported to give good pain relief in 80% of patients (Paech, 2000). For these reasons low dose epidural local anaesthetic and opioid mixtures such as 0.1–0.125% bupivacaine is usually used with either fentanyl 2–5 µg/ml, pethidine 2.5 mg/ml, or diamorphine 0.25 mg/ml.

BENEFICIAL EFFECTS OF EPIDURALS FOR THE MOTHER

Pain causes a stress response during which the body produces catecholamines, adrenaline and noradrenaline into the circulation; these substances improve the body's ability to deal with pain by increasing the heart rate and improving blood flow to contracting muscles. However, during labour adrenaline can diminish the strength and synchrony of the uterine contractions and an uncoordinated labour may ensue. So an epidural infusion can reduce pain, reduce the body's stress response and assist with a more coordinated and effective labour.

The stress response and excessive amounts of catecholamines can also cause hyperventilation resulting in an imbalance of the mother's acid–base balance (pH) reducing the delivery of oxygen to the baby. An epidural has been demonstrated to be beneficial in labour as it normalises the levels of catecholamines and regulates the mother's breathing pattern as the pain reduces and relaxation is possible.

ADVERSE EFFECTS OF EPIDURALS FOR THE MOTHER

For general information on adverse effects associated with local anaesthetic and opioid administration see Chapter 4.

Respiratory Depression

Clinically significant maternal respiratory depression can occur although it is relatively rare, estimated to be approximately 1 in 5000 cases (Hughes, 1997), therefore appropriate close monitoring is mandatory. However, pregnant women are thought to be at a lower risk of respiratory depression than their non-pregnant counterparts because they are mainly healthy patients with a protective mechanism relating to the respiratory stimulant effects of progesterone (Paech, 2000).

During labour hypoxic episodes often occur in women experiencing painful labour (particularly if they are obese). Hypoventilation can occur during a painful contraction and desaturation often follows. Epidural analgesia is beneficial because it helps to alleviate this situation (Paech, 2000).

Hypotension

The local anaesthetic that is injected into the epidural space has the potential to block all nerves that it comes into contact with, not just the A delta and C fibres which are responsible for pain transmission. It may also affect nerves that are involved with muscle power, tone of blood vessels and blood pressure control. Such hypotensive effects of local anaesthetics are in general dose related.

A fall in blood pressure invariably occurs in labour after the mother receives an epidural because the blood pressure is often high due to pain prior to catheter insertion. As the pain subsides so the blood pressure begins to fall back to normal levels. Hypotension also occurs because the epidural relaxes the muscles in the walls of the blood vessels, which were previously constricted secondary to pain. As vasodilation occurs so does a fall in blood pressure.

An intravenous cannula should be inserted prior to commencement of the epidural infusion so that intravenous therapy can be commenced to compensate for any hypotensive effects. If the blood pressure does not respond it may require the addition of a vasopressor drug such as ephedrine, which causes the blood vessels to constrict.

Supine Hypotension

Lying flat for any length of time during the end stages of pregnancy is harmful because it interferes with general circulation. The weight of the baby compresses the aorta and vena cava, which lie directly in front of the spine. Compression of the aorta can severely restrict blood flow to the legs, to some major organs and also to the uterus. If this is prolonged for more than a few minutes it can interfere with the oxygen supply to the baby. Compression of the vena cava also interferes with blood flow returning to the heart causing the mother to have a fall in blood pressure, feel faint, light-headed and nauseous. It is important to avoid these symptoms by ensuring that pregnant women are not allowed to lie flat.

Pruritus

Pregnancy appears to increase the risk of pruritus possibly due to altered opioid receptor binding competition relating to oestrogen levels, higher endogenous opioid levels and greater cephalic spread. Fentanyl has a lower incidence for pruritus than morphine.

Nausea and Vomiting

In labour nausea and vomiting are common irrespective of pain relief and are not directly related to gastrointestinal stasis, physiological effects of pain stimulation or effects of the opioid drugs. Epidural analgesia does not appear to increase the risk of nausea and vomiting.

Urinary Retention

Both local anaesthetics and opioids can increase the risk of urinary retention. Muscle weakness associated with the epidurals has the potential to cause the bladder to become overfull. The use of dilute local anaesthetic solutions can help to preserve bladder sensation although it may be necessary for the midwife to temporarily catheterise the mother. Post-delivery there are some clear data that suggest that for some women there will be a residual loss of bladder function which is not associated with an increased incidence in patients who had epidural pain relief in labour. With caesarean section approximately 50% of women will suffer acute urinary retention, after vaginal delivery approximately 2–18% of patients will suffer urinary retention (Paech, 2000). Prolonged secondary stage of labour also increases the risk.

Motor Block

Local anaesthetics can cause some numbness and weakness in the legs causing decreased control over movement and the ability to stand. The extent of the motor block depends largely on the strength and quantity of the local anaesthetic given. Monitoring of motor block is essential if pressure sores and accidental falls are to be avoided.

Nerve Injury

Occasionally some temporary damage may occur to peripheral nerves during delivery of the baby as a result of direct pressure from the baby's head or from direct injury from instrumentation like forceps or epidural catheter insertion. The incidence of such nerve injury is no higher in epidural patients than in those who receive other types of analgesia. Signs of nerve injury include numbness, weakness and/or pain, also some bladder and anal sphincter disturbance can occur. Of these problems 99% will be spontaneously resolved; permanent paralysis resulting directly from epidural insertion is extremely rare.

Epidurals and Long-term Backache

Reports that increased motor block is associated with long-term backache after delivery are unfounded (Paech, 2000). Postural backache is common in pregnancy with an estimated 50% of women suffering at some time during their pregnancy. Some women complain of post-delivery back pain that is likely to be musculoskeletal in origin. Insertion of an epidural catheter can cause some tenderness at the entry site, but this usually resolves spontaneously within a few days. Pain can also be associated with lumbar lordosis and joint laxity from elevated levels of hormones (Paech, 2000). Generally the more severe the back pain during pregnancy the longer it lasts post-delivery.

Suggestions have been made that there could be a potential connection between epidural analgesia in labour and post-delivery back pain. It may be that during the pain free state when the epidural infusion is in progress muscular relaxation occurs resulting in postural backache. Two British studies associate the provision of epidural analgesia during labour with new long-term backache (Russell *et al.*, 1993; MacArthur *et al.*, 1995). These studies were

Table 6.1. Studies showing no direct connection between epidural catheter placement and long-term back pain

Study	Type of study	Number of patients	Incidence of new back pain with epidural (%)	Incidence of new back pain without epidural (%)
Breen *et al.*, 1994	Prospective observational	1042	44	45
MacArthur *et al.*, 1995	Prospective cohort study follow up at 1 year	244	10	14
Patel *et al.*, 1995	Prospective 6–8 months postpartum	340	7	6
Russell *et al.*, 1996	Prospective randomised controlled trial 1 year postpartum	450	No difference between groups	No difference between groups
Loughnan *et al.*, 1997	Prospective randomised controlled trial 6 months postpartum	409	32	28
Breen *et al.*, 1999	Prospective randomised controlled trial 6 months postpartum	93 (27 at 6 months)	27	33

retrospective and respondent rates were low, also there are questions raised regarding the accuracy of response recall with some questionnaires being distributed up to eight years post-delivery, potentially causing some bias in the study results.

There is a plethora of studies that dispute the connection between epidural analgesia and back pain (Table 6.1). There is also growing evidence to suggest that back pain following epidural catheter placement is no more common than after other forms of analgesia.

Epidurals and Headache

The distance across the epidural space is very small, if the epidural needle is pushed a little too far it may pierce the dura, which forms the spinal sac and contains the cerebrospinal fluid (CSF). Accidental puncture of the dura during placement of the epidural catheter can lead to a leakage of CSF into the epidural space and a loss of pressure around the brain and spinal cord which manifests itself as a 'post-dural puncture headache' (PDPH). It should, however, be noted that headache following delivery is not uncommon regardless of analgesic technique.

This type of headache usually develops within 18 hours of the puncture and lasts for four to five days. It is felt both in the head and the back of the neck and is classified by its postural nature; it is exacerbated by standing upright and to a greater extent with mobilisation. It may be associated with audio or visual symptoms, which usually develop 24 hours after the dural puncture occurs. The smaller the needle that causes the puncture and the smaller the puncture itself the less severe the headache tends to be.

Dehydration may exacerbate the headache, so it is important to keep the patient well hydrated once a PDPH is diagnosed. Simple analgesics can help but are often not sufficient to control the headache. Cerebrovasoconstrictors (e.g. caffeine) can be given with some success and often the symptoms will subside spontaneously. Where the headache is particularly severe or fails to subside it may be necessary to carry out a blood patch.

Epidural Blood Patch

This technique involves a slow epidural injection of approximately 20 ml of autologous blood (at the same epidural level as the epidural was performed) in an attempt to close the hole in the dura, stop the leakage of CSF and cure the PDPH. Following administration of the blood a small amount of saline should be injected to minimise the risk of backtracking of blood into the soft tissues causing a haematoma and further problems with back pain. To maximise the effect the patient should rest for a few hours and then mobilise very slowly post-injection. This procedure although generally effective does carry a small risk of repeat dural puncture, which should be explained to the patient.

BENEFICIAL EFFECTS OF EPIDURALS ON THE BABY

A mother who is experiencing severe pain in labour may initiate a physiological stress response, which can interfere with the normal progress of labour and in turn can increase the stress levels of the baby. Stress can be monitored in the baby in a number of ways including recording the baby's heart rate, a cardiotacograph trace or the appearance of meconium. A technique such as an epidural, which reduces the mother's stress during labour, will be of benefit to the baby.

ADVERSE EFFECTS OF EPIDURALS FOR THE BABY

Hypoxia

A baby whose mother has a significant hypotensive event can become hypoxic because there is a decrease in the flow of blood and therefore oxygen to the placenta. It should, however, be remembered that although local anaesthetic may cause some degree of hypotension other causes should also be considered.

The delivery of oxygen to the baby is determined by the concentration of oxygen in the mother's blood and the blood flow to the placenta. Hypoxia can occur if the mother is heavily sedated by excessive opioid doses.

Drug toxicity

After administration of opioids the maternal drug distribution is rapid and problems are most likely to occur when the fetal blood concentrations are at their peak (fetal aortic flow increases during labour but decreases with narcotic agents). Morphine and pethidine freely cross the placenta (as do all opioid drugs) and umbilical venous blood concentrations have been shown to be similar to that of maternal blood within two minutes of an intravenous injection. The depressant effects of the blood concentration are greater in the neonate than in the mother perhaps due to an immature respiratory centre or because the placenta acts as a store for lipid soluble opioids. Epidurals allow very small doses of opioids to be administered reducing the risks outlined.

Epidural administration of low dose opioids is a relatively safe option for the baby as very low or undetectable umbilical venous and arterial levels of opioids have been reported. Fentanyl is often the drug of choice and although it does not have an adverse effect on the baby's heart rate variability, Apgar scores and umbilical blood gas values, it does not depress neonatal respiration, alter respiratory parameters or patterns of breathing, nor does it affect neurobehaviour (Paech, 2000).

Local anaesthetics can affect the baby indirectly by blocking sympathetic activity causing hypotension in the mother or directly by crossing the placental barrier and reducing placental blood flow (Harmer, 1997). Fetal local anaesthetic levels rise with increasing maternal administration and severe fetal adverse effects are only likely to be seen at maternal toxic doses (Paech, 2000). Bupivacaine is usually the local anaesthetic of choice because it is relatively long acting with minimal plasma accumulation and transfer across the placental barrier (Moir, 1982).

POST-CAESAREAN SECTION ANALGESIA

Epidurals not only provide excellent pain management during labour, they can also be utilised postoperatively once caesarean section has taken place. Most obstetric patients are healthy, well motivated and desire good pain relief so epidural analgesia is ideal. Again either continuous or patient controlled epidural analgesia (PCEA) delivery systems can be used. PCEA significantly reduces drug consumption and therefore associated unwanted side effects particularly in breastfeeding mothers.

REFERENCES

Association of Anaesthetists of Great Britain and Ireland and the Obstetric Anaesthetists Association (1998) *Guidelines for Obstetric Anaesthesia Services*. Hampshire: Alresford Press.

Beavis, R. (1984) *Anaesthesia in Midwifery*. London: Baillière Tindall.

Breen, T. (1996) Optimal labour analgesia. *Canadian Journal of Anesthesia*, **90**, 944–50.

Breen, T., Ransil, B., Groves, P. and Oriol, N. (1994) Factors associated with back pain after childbirth. *Anaesthesiology*, **81**, 29–34.

Breen, T., Campbell, M., Halpern, S. *et al.* (1999) Epidural analgesia and back pain following delivery: a prospective randomised study. *Anaesthesiology*, **90**, A7.

Brownridge, P. (1991) Epidural analgesia in the first stage of labour. *Anaesthesia and Critical Care*, **2**, 92–100.

Clarke, A., Carr, D., Loyd, G. *et al.* (1998) The influence of epidural analgesia on caesarean delivery rates: a randomised prospective clinical trail. *American Journal of Obstetrics and Gynecology*, **179**, 1527–33.

Collis, R., Davies, D. and Aveling, W. (1995) Randomised comparisons of combined spinal-epidural and standard epidural analgesia in labour. *Lancet*, **345**, 1413–6.

Gambling, D., McMorland, G., Yu, P. and Laszio, C. (1990) Comparison of patient controlled epidural analgesia and conventional intermittent top-up injections during labour. *Anesthesia & Analgesia*, **70**, 256–61.

Halpern, S., Leighton, B., Ohisson, A. *et al.* (1998) Effect of epidural vs parenteral opioid analgesia on the progress of labour. A meta-analysis. *JAMA*, **280**, 2105–10.

Harmer, M. (1997) *Pain in Obstetrics and Gynaecology*. Module Nine MSc in Pain Management. Cardiff: UWCM.

Howell, C. (2004) Epidural versus non-epidural analgesia for pain relief in labour (Cochrane review) In: *The Cochrane Library*, Issue 2. Chichester: John Wiley & Sons.

Hughes, S. (1997) Respiratory depression following intra-spinal narcotics: expect it! *International Journal of Obstetrics and Anaesthesia*, **6**, 145–6.

Loughnan, B., Carli, R., Romney, M. *et al.* (1997) The influence of epidural analgesia on the development of new backache in primiparous women: report of a randomised controlled trial. *International Journal of Obstetrics and Anaesthesia*, **6**, 203–4.

MacArthur, A., MacArthur, C. and Weeks, S. (1995) Epidural anaesthesia and long-term back pain after delivery: a prospective cohort study. *British Medical Journal*, **311**, 1336–9.

Moir, D. (1982) *Pain Relief in Labour*, 4th edn. New York: Churchill Livingstone.

Paech, M. (2000) Regional analgesia and anaesthesia. In: Russell, R. (ed.). *Anaesthesia for Obstetrics and Gynaecology*. London: British Medical Journal Publishing Group.

Patel, M., Fernando, R., Gill, P. *et al.* (1995) A prospective study of long-term backache after childbirth in primigravidae – the effect of ambulatory epidural analgesia during labour. *International Journal of Obstetric Anaesthesia*, **4**, 187.

Royal College of Anaesthetists (2001) *Pain Relief in Labour*, 2nd edn. London: Obstetric Anaesthetists Association.

Royal College of Anaesthetists and Association of Anaesthetists of Great Britain and Ireland (2004) *Epidural for Pain Relief After Surgery*. London: RCA/AAGBI.

Royal College of Anaesthetists, Royal College of Nursing, Association of Anaesthetists of Great Britain and Ireland, the British Pain Society and the European Society of Regional Anaesthesia and Pain Therapy (2004) *Good Practice in the Management of Continuous Epidural Analgesia in the Hospital Setting*. London: RCA.

Russell, R., Groves, P., Taub, N. *et al.* (1993) Assessing long term backache after childbirth. *British Medical Journal*, **306**, 1299–302.

Russell, R., Dundas, R. and Reynolds, F. (1996) Long-term backache after childbirth: prospective search for causative factors. *British Medical Journal*, **312**, 1384–8.

Russell, R., Scrutton, M. and Porter, J. (1997) *Pain Relief in Labour*. London: British Medical Journal Publishing Group.

Scott, W. (1991) Ethics in obstetric analgesia. *Anaesthesia*, **51**, 717–8.

Steer, P. (1993) The availability of pain relief. In: Chamberlain, G., Wraight, A. and Steer, P. (eds) *Pain and its Relief in Childbirth*. New York: Churchill Livingstone.

7

Epidurals in Paediatric Practice

CAROLYN MIDDLETON
Clinical Nurse Specialist in Pain Management, Nevill Hall Hospital,
Abergavenny, South Wales

For physiological and humanitarian reasons pain should be safely and effectively managed in all age groups. However, there is evidence that this has not always been the case for babies and young children (Grundy *et al.*, 1993). It is likely that this is due predominantly to clinicians lacking both knowledge and the confidence to administer appropriate doses of analgesia to paediatric patients because of the associated potential side effects.

The aim of this chapter is to provide an overview of the differences between paediatric and adult pain transmission; to explore the specific issues relating to the pharmacokinetics and pharmacodynamics of epidural drugs in paediatric patients; and to review the provision of paediatric pain services, issues surrounding consent for minors and special precautions relating to epidural catheter insertion in children.

PAEDIATRIC PAIN TRANSMISSION

The neurobiology of pain following tissue damage in children is well documented; it is similar to the neurobiology of adults and is reliant upon action potentials to transmit nociceptive information from the periphery via the dorsal horn to the brain (Chapter 4). The absence of full myelination in the neonatal and infant nervous system is a reflection of immaturity and not an

Epidural Analgesia in Acute Pain Management. Edited by Carolyn Middleton.
© 2006 by John Wiley & Sons, Ltd.   ISBN 0-470-01964-6

indication of lack of function in pain processing, therefore children of all ages are capable of experiencing pain.

However, there are important functional differences between adults and children in pain processing. Firstly, the receptive fields of individual neurones are much larger in children, therefore younger patients experience greater difficulty in localising pain accurately (Yu and Barr, 1995). Secondly, activity in non-nociceptive fibres Aalpha and Abeta in very young babies can activate neurones in the dorsal horn that are predominantly nociceptive in adults. This suggests that babies and very young children may actually experience more pain than older children and adults (Jennings and Fitzgerald, 1996). Thirdly, there are differences in the proportion of opioid receptors in neonates, which may contribute to their reduced ability to modulate nociceptive transmission and once again cause an increase in pain sensation (Jennings and Fitzgerald, 1996).

Finally, there is also evidence that the descending inhibitory pathways may be less well developed in younger patients than in adults. This may contribute to a reduced ability to modulate nociceptive transmission with techniques such as the production of naturally occurring endorphin analgesics; this can only add to the child's pain experience (Kar and Quirion, 1995). Therefore, careful attention to pain control should be a part of every child's post-trauma or post-operative management.

PAEDIATRIC PAIN SERVICE AND EPIDURAL PROVISION

The Royal College of Anaesthetists (2001) recommends that where paediatric epidurals are being used there is need for a comprehensive, quality service dedicated to the care of paediatric patients and to the education and development of staff. This provision must include paediatric trained anaesthetic staff and should be led by a consultant anaesthetist who regularly anaesthetises children. There should also be a dedicated acute pain team on site whose remit includes overseeing all clinical and educational aspects of a paediatric epidural service. Also a pain team member should visit all children with an epidural catheter in place at least once per day to ensure safe and effective analgesic delivery.

It is important that parents or carers of children receiving epidural analgesia should be involved in all aspects of the care and decision making regarding their child (RCA, 2001). Parents and children should receive written and verbal preoperative information that outlines the epidural procedure, risks and benefits involved and there should be documented evidence that these issues have been discussed. Both parents and health professionals should be involved in the psychological and physical preparation of a child who is to receive epidural analgesia.

Post-insertion of an epidural catheter, each child should be nursed on a ward where there are at least two registered children's nurses on duty for every shift that the child is present (RCA, 2001). There should also be a high dependency unit available if required for the immediate period post-insertion of an epidural; the need for this would usually be determined by the extent of the trauma sustained or the surgical procedure undergone.

CONSENT

General issues relating to consent have been outlined in Chapter 2, but there are some specific issues relating to paediatric practice. In English law young people aged between 16 and 17 years can give consent to treatment without their decision being referred to their parents or guardians, although as a matter of good practice an anaesthetist might wish to involve the parents, but parents cannot overrule a young person's decision to give consent.

Children under 16 years who understand what is proposed can give consent to medical interventions such as insertion of an epidural catheter. The anaesthetist must judge whether or not the individual child has the maturity to fully comprehend the issues relating to the procedure, the risks, benefits and alternatives available. If so the child is deemed to be competent and again in these circumstances the parents cannot overrule the child's decision.

Unless a child under 16 years old is deemed to be competent, the anaesthetists must obtain consent from parents or guardians who are legally and morally entitled to give or withhold consent. Their decision will usually be upheld unless it conflicts seriously with the anaesthetist's views on the child's best interests. The law says that best interests and the balance of benefits and burdens are essential components of the decision-making process (Chapter 2) and that the views of the parents form only part of this. If agreement cannot be reached legal review may be required.

Best practice suggests that children should be involved in the decision-making process whenever possible and appropriate.

PRIOR TO INSERTION OF EPIDURAL CATHETER

Topical application of local anaesthetic to the skin to provide cutaneous anaesthesia for all children over one month old should be routine practice prior to all needling procedures associated with epidural catheter insertion (Arrowsmith and Campbell, 2000). The eutectic mixture of local anaesthetics prilocaine and lignocaine (EMLA cream) or amethocaine gel (4%) are most commonly used. Amethocaine has the advantage of a more rapid onset time of 30 minutes (Dunnett, 1996), whereas EMLA requires one hour for a reliable response (Arendt-Nielsen and Bjerring, 1988).

EPIDURAL CATHETER INSERTION

All aspects of insertion techniques are similar to those described in Chapter 3, but it is normal practice for epidural catheters to be sited in children after induction of anaesthesia. This is done because it is technically more difficult to site an epidural catheter in a young child who cannot keep completely still, it is also less distressing for the child to have the procedure carried out while asleep.

The technique to identify loss of resistance can involve using a burette and giving set primed with saline (rather than a loss of resistance syringe – see Chapter 3) which is attached to the Tuohy needle. Observation of commencement of droplets of saline advancing from the burette provides identification that the needle has passed through the ligamentum flavum and is in fact in the epidural space.

Preventing inadvertent dural puncture during advancement of the Tuohy needle requires a careful technique with a half-length paediatric 18g needle for small infants as the extradural space in neonates and infants may be as little as 5mm from the skin (Hassan *et al.*, 1994; Bosenberg, 1995). Although dural puncture should be relatively rare, when it does occur in paediatric patients persistent cerebrospinal fluid (CSF) leakage may present with symptoms including nausea and dizziness (McHale and O'Donovan, 1997). Treatment for post-dural puncture headache may require treatment with an epidural blood patch.

As children tend to be far more mobile postoperatively than adults there is a greater risk of kinking or occlusion of the epidural catheter, particularly where single end hole catheters are used (Figure 7.1). Multiple fenestration catheters tend to be less prone to these problems and are therefore more appropriate for use in younger children (Wilson and Lloyd-Thomas, 1993; Lloyd-Thomas and Howard, 1994; Woolf, 1994).

EPIDURAL DRUGS

LOCAL ANAESTHETICS

General information regarding the use of epidural local anaesthetics has been discussed in Chapter 3; there is evidence that this class of drugs is an essential component in the control of movement induced pain (Dahl *et al.*, 1992). There are nevertheless specific problems related to using this class of drugs for

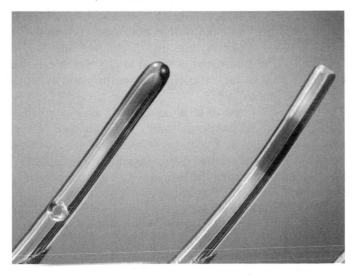

Figure 7.1. End and multiple fenestration epidural catheters. (Reproduced by permission of B-Braun Medical Ltd.)

paediatric patients: the metabolic half-life of local anaesthetics is longer in neonates and infants than in adults, therefore there is concern regarding the ability of very young children to metabolise and clear amide local anaesthetic drugs compared with older children or adults (Eyres, 1995). This prolonged half-life of local anaesthetic drugs renders babies particularly susceptible to the side effects of these drugs.

There have been several reports of toxicity from local anaesthetics especially when they are given by continuous infusion as accumulation can occur, although high doses of local anaesthetics were used in some of these reports (Ved *et al.*, 1993; Larsson *et al.*, 1994; Maxwell *et al.*, 1994). The toxicity of a local anaesthetic drug is dependent upon the rate of rise of plasma local anaesthetic concentration, the protein binding of local anaesthetic agent, the concurrent use of central nervous system depressants and the immaturity of the blood–brain barrier (Eyres, 1995). It is clear that these drugs need to be used with care in the very young, consequently minimal doses of local anaesthetics should be used to ensure the lowest risk of toxicity along with careful dose titration when infusions are used (Cheung *et al.*, 1997; Peutrell *et al.*, 1997). Adult dose recommendations are based on the results of clinical trials but with a lack of such studies using paediatric patients, body weight and height are usually used as a basis for paediatric dose calculation.

Toxicity from local anaesthetic drugs has already been discussed in Chapter 4. In paediatric patients the cardio-vascular system (CVS) symptom of collapse may be the first sign of local anaesthetic toxicity, thus basic life support equipment and expertise must be available as a precaution (Maxwell *et al.*, 1994). Central nervous system symptoms in children include somnolence, heaviness of the head and impaired postural ability which can then progress to paraesthesia, tinnitus, visual disturbance, dysarthria and eventually convulsions (Peutrell and Hughes, 1995).

In order to minimise the risk of local anaesthetic toxicity epidural catheters should be sited adjacent to the dermatomes to be blocked (Chapter 3), this allows lower concentrations and volumes of local anaesthetic to be infused to produce excellent analgesic results. Compensating for a catheter that is less than ideally placed by increasing the infusion rate is hazardous (Berde, 1994).

The use of bupivacaine alone may cause problems in infants despite the provision of excellent analgesia because of the lack of sedation. This may be provided by small amounts of opioid added to the epidural solution.

OPIOIDS

General information regarding the use of epidural opioids has been discussed in Chapter 3. In paediatric practice morphine, diamorphine and fentanyl are the opioids most studied but it must be noted that the pharmacokinetics of opioid drugs alters with age (Wilson and Lloyd-Thomas, 1993; Wood *et al.*, 1994). Protein binding is reduced in infancy and the neonatal period with an increase in free drug available in plasma to bind to opioid receptors (Bhat *et al.*, 1990; McRorie *et al.*, 1992).

The lipid solubility of the chosen drug affects the dose required, the speed of onset, the duration of action and the degree of complications. Fentanyl is a highly lipid soluble drug so it will have a rapid transfer across the dura to the opioid receptor sites and therefore a quicker onset of analgesia. But the duration of action is shorter as the drug will be removed more quickly from receptor sites by blood flow.

Morphine is a relatively low lipid soluble drug so it will take longer to act and stays for a greater length of time in the CSF. This has implications with regard to spread of the drug away from the point of injection, the drug may be carried by the CSF circulation upwards towards the brain and cause unwanted side effects such as respiratory depression (with more lipid soluble drugs like fentanyl a greater proportion of the dose is absorbed systemically and this problem is less likely to occur). Respiratory depression in paediatric patients receiving epidural opioids is rare with an incidence reported to be less than 1% (Henneberg *et al.*, 1993; Lloyd-Thomas and Howard, 1994). However, mild respiratory slowing and sedation are more commonly seen with approximately 6.5% of children affected (Lloyd-Thomas and Howard, 1994).

Morphine usage in very young children tends to be somewhat unpredictable. The half-life is prolonged, the volume of distribution is increased and the clearance is reduced (Hartley and Levene, 1995). There are also significant inter-patient differences in morphine metabolism; a mature, healthy term neonate of two weeks of age may have morphine metabolism, clearance and half-life figures similar to an adult, while another infant of six weeks of age may still have immature metabolism and a long half-life. Therefore the likelihood of side effects related to epidural opioids is increased.

In older children urinary retention is a particular problem (Lloyd-Thomas and Howard, 1994). Restricting the opioid dose, ensuring adequate post-operative fluids, using naloxone at small doses (0.5 µg/kg) and elective urinary catheterisation at the time of operation will minimise the impact of this side effect (Lloyd-Thomas, 1993; Berde, 1994).

Despite these problems in paediatric practice, the addition of an opioid to an epidural infusion can enhance the quality of analgesia without the sympathetic or motor blockade sometimes seen when local anaesthetics are used in isolation. On safety grounds the highly lipid soluble drug fentanyl is often the drug of choice.

ADVERSE DRUG REACTIONS

As any technique increases in popularity and numbers rise, complications associated with treatment will be seen more frequently (Dunwoody *et al.*, 1997; Larsson *et al.*, 1994; McHale and O'Donovan, 1997; Meunier *et al.*, 1997). However, carefully conducted epidural analgesia is safe and effective (Giaufre *et al*, 1996). For detailed information relating to side effects of epidural analgesia and their management see Chapter 10, but a brief overview of problems associated with paediatric epidural will be given here.

The incidence of opioid induced respiratory depression is reported to be less than 1% (Henneberg *et al.*, 1993; Lloyd-Thomas and Howard, 1994). However, mild respiratory slowing and sedation are more commonly seen with approximately 6.5% of children affected (Lloyd-Thomas and Howard, 1994). This effect can be reversed by incremental administration of the opioid antagonist naloxone.

Nausea and vomiting are also opioid induced. The incidence is low in young patients with approximately 2% of infants affected; this rate rises to between 30% and 50% in children over 10 years of age (Lloyd-Thomas and Howard, 1994). Using balanced analgesia can help to reduce the associated side effects as can administration of the antiemetic ondansetron which appears to be highly effective.

Opioids and local anaesthetics can inhibit the micturition reflex causing urinary retention in up to 30% of children, catheterisation is often needed and many anaesthetists will do this prophylactically in any child receiving epidural.

Lack of lower limb sensation and the potential to develop pressure sores may cause problems, therefore motor block must be assessed regularly. Where a dense block does exist infusion rates should be reduced and patients repositioned regularly.

Issues relating to hypotension, pruritis, haematoma, infection, hallucinations and headache have a similar incidence and treatment management regimen to adults, and information is provided in Chapter 10.

The use of epidural infusion or intermittent top-ups in the postoperative period requires close nursing supervision of the child in order to detect any of these potential complications, which if detected should be acted on appropriately.

DRUG DELIVERY SYSTEMS

INTERMITTENT VERSUS CONTINUOUS ADMINISTRATION

As soon as continuous infusion techniques are introduced into paediatric analgesia practice there are risks and benefits to be balanced (Chapter 5). All paediatric infusions should be regarded as high risk and must therefore be closely monitored by appropriately trained staff.

Good quality analgesia is more likely to be provided with a continuous infusion than with intermittent top-up dosing. Plasma concentrations of bupivacaine during continuous epidural infusions must be significantly below toxicity levels, however accumulation of total and free bupivacaine has been reported in neonates. The minimum effective dose must be used and significantly lower hourly dosages should be given to neonates than to other paediatric patients.

If undesirable (but not life threatening) side effects are a problem with continuous delivery of epidural solution the infusion needs to be turned off until the side effects have been resolved. The infusion can then be resumed at a lower dose, usually about 50% of the previous dose.

PCEA

Sophisticated microprocessor controlled electronic pumps have allowed the introduction of patient controlled epidural analgesia (PCEA) for children (Bray *et al.*, 1996). These pumps are capable of delivering accurate bolus doses on demand, thus titrating epidural solution delivery against the patient's level of pain.

Patient controlled analgesia has been shown to be safe and effective in children as young as seven years of age. PCEA allows for variation in analgesic requirement between patients and in the same patient over time. It also gives a child control over his or her own analgesia, which has considerable psychological benefits. PCEA is often most effective with a small continuous infusion rate alongside the patient control system.

The decision to allow the self-delivery of supplementary doses requires careful assessment of each individual child, the child must be able to understand the basic concept of PCEA and have the dexterity to operate the demand button (Lloyd-Thomas and Howard, 1994). PCEA is definitely unsuitable for children with physical disabilities or severe injuries involving the hands, children who are unwilling to use the device or those with a lack of mental capacity to understand the concept of PCEA.

Patients using the PCEA system will require considerable preoperative preparation and postoperative support (Lloyd-Thomas and Howard, 1994). Conversion to continuous only infusion should be undertaken if there is doubt as to the competence of the patient postoperatively and parents should always be instructed never to give doses on their child's behalf as pain stimulates respiratory function and administration of demand doses to a well analgesed child increases the risk of respiratory depression. Monitoring for PCEA patients has to be at least as intensive as that for conventional epidural infusion (Chapter 8).

CO-PRESCRIBING

There are other medications that should be co-prescribed alongside the epidural infusion, these include an opioid antagonist, oxygen, balanced analgesia and an appropriate antiemetic.

Naloxone

Naloxone, a synthetic opioid antagonist, should always be prescribed whenever an opioid is being administered. Naloxone reverses the respiratory depressive effects of the opioid (Chapter 4). The recommended intravenous dose for paediatric patients is 10 μg/kg body weight.

The half-life of naloxone is shorter than the half-life of the opioid, so the effects will wear off while the opioid is still active putting the patient at further risk of respiratory depression.

Oxygen

Oxygen should also be prescribed to paediatric patients who receive epidural analgesia. The potential respiratory problem coupled with the potential for opioid induced respiratory depression means that careful monitoring of oxygen saturation levels and respiratory activities is essential (Chapter 8).

Balanced Analgesia

The increased understanding of pain transmission has underlined a need to use a wide spectrum of analgesic medications simultaneously for optimal pain management; this is the concept of 'balanced analgesia' (Kehlet, 1994). A balanced technique of analgesia uses drugs that modify nociceptive transmission at different points in the pain pathway as per the World Health Organisation analgesic ladder (Chapter 4).

Non-steroidal Anti-inflammatory Drugs (NSAIDs)

NSAIDs are now widely used for postoperative analgesia in children following major surgery and convenient syrup, suppository and 'melt' formulations are available. The well recognised contraindications to these drugs must be carefully observed, however pre-existing pathology, such as gastrointestinal adverse effects, is most commonly seen in adults and much less common in children.

There is a specific caution with NSAIDs in paediatric patients as the incidence of asthma is increasing, although many asthmatics will be able to tolerate NSAIDs with no adverse reaction. It is probably unwise to use these drugs in infants as renal maturation is still occurring in the first year of life.

Paracetamol

Paracetamol is very convenient and effective in children when given as a co-analgesic in adequate doses; it has been described as the cornerstone of paediatric analgesic management. It too is available in tablet, syrup, rectal suppository and intravenous formulations.

The absorption from the rectal route is slow and it is now realised that higher loading doses up to 40mg/kg are required to achieve therapeutic plasma concentrations with subsequent maintenance doses. The maximum recommended dose of paracetamol (regardless of route of administration) is 90mg/kg per day (Southall, 1997). Oral paracetamol premedication is useful in establishing a therapeutic plasma concentration in time for recovery.

Balanced analgesia does not only imply the use of medication, but will also use the skills of nurses and parents in distraction techniques and other forms of comfort therapy.

Step-down Analgesia

Step-down analgesia should be put into place once a decision is made to discontinue the epidural. This should be done adhering to the World Health Organisation analgesic ladder and stepping down from the top of the ladder (severe pain – strong opioid + NSAID + simple analgesic agent) to the middle of the ladder (moderate pain – weak opioid + NSAID + simple analgesic agent). First dosing of the step-down analgesic agents should occur approximately 30 minutes prior to the epidural being discontinued so that the oral analgesia begins to exert an effect when the epidural is stopped.

NON-PHARMACOLOGICAL ADJUNCTS

The emotional component of pain must also be addressed in all aspects of paediatric practice using instinctive comforting measures, provision of child friendly surroundings, distraction techniques and giving the child and family the chance to be involved and in control of their pain management. These non-pharmacological techniques should be used to complement safe and effective use of analgesic drugs.

MONITORING

Development of minimum monitoring standards for all children receiving complex techniques such as epidural infusion is essential. Suitably trained qualified staff should provide the monitoring.

Children must be carefully matched to the technique, level of expertise and available facilities for monitoring, with neonates requiring special care because of the differences in opioid and local anaesthetic pharmacology. The currently recommended monitoring standard comprises regular (preferably hourly) assessments of analgesic efficacy, of adverse effects and of the infusion system. Further information regarding observation monitoring can be found in Chapter 8.

Pain Assessment

Poor pain assessment in children has been one possible reason for inadequate analgesia being delivered (Hester, 1995). Paediatric pain assessment must be practical to perform and must track both the pain experience of the child and the efficacy of analgesic interventions over time. The assessment has to be appropriate for the child's stage of development and the surgical procedure undertaken. Pain verbalisation ability changes with age so a great deal of work has been done to develop both behavioural observation tools for the very young and paediatric self-reporting scales for slightly older children (Kiechel and Bildner, 1995; Sparshott, 1996).

Wherever possible the tool chosen should combine the child's self-report with the child's and health professionals' assessment. This is not possible in the very young, so in order to pick up the signs of pain behavioural cues and physiological values are used. In neonates, scoring systems such as the CRIES tool can be used. This has a scoring system from 0 to 2 and measures the child's crying, facial expressions, movement, physiology (i.e. blood pressure and heart rate), oxygen requirements and oxygen saturation levels. Higher scores indicate increased pain levels. This tool is relatively easy to use and works well in all but very preterm babies.

In infants and toddlers (aged 1 to 5 years) the Toddler Preschool Postoperative Pain Scale (TPPPS) has been found to be a useful. Once again a 0 to 2 scoring system is used against the following parameters: verbal expression, facial expression, posture, movement and physiology. Again the higher the score the greater the pain intensity.

The major problems with these scoring systems are: firstly, that specificity of respiratory and cardiovascular responses tends to be low because measures of oxygenation will be influenced by underlying pulmonary or cardiac pathology (McGrath *et al.*, 1987); secondly, it must be remembered that cry cannot be estimated in intubated patients receiving respiratory support; finally, it should be noted that facial expression changes with age potentially underestimating postoperative pain behaviour, so caution is required in the use of these scoring systems (Craig, 1992). However, if these tools are used with care and their limitations are realised, they can significantly assist with objective assessment of paediatric pain (Tyler *et al.*, 1993).

From three years of age children can self-report the presence and intensity of pain. Self-reporting, with the use of visual aids such as the smiley faces, is the most accurate method of pain assessment (Figure 7.2).

From seven years of age a visual analogue scale (VAS) can be used where the child scores his or her pain on a horizontal line with or without associated numerical calibrations (Chapter 8).

Whichever scoring system is used, pain assessment should not be carried out in isolation; it should be linked to appropriate interventions with the aim of

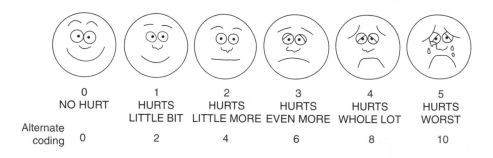
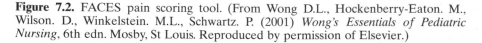

Figure 7.2. FACES pain scoring tool. (From Wong D.L., Hockenberry-Eaton. M., Wilson. D., Winkelstein. M.L., Schwartz. P. (2001) *Wong's Essentials of Pediatric Nursing*, 6th edn. Mosby, St Louis. Reproduced by permission of Elsevier.)

ensuring the child's comfort. The assessments should be carried out on movement rather than at rest, as pain-free movement and return to normal functioning along with the ability to co-operate with physiotherapy are the aims of good analgesia management. If this is not done, there is a risk of the child lying rigidly still, afraid to move, cough or breath deeply and being scored as having 'no pain'.

Most paediatric pain can be prevented or controlled by proven safe and effective measures such as epidural infusion. Coordination of analgesic management by dedicated multidisciplinary pain teams is the best way to achieve a comprehensive provision of safe pain control for all children.

TECHNICAL PROBLEMS

Technical problems with the equipment are not uncommon when epidural infusions are used in children, as children tend to be far more mobile in bed than adult patients. The problems that do occur include obstruction of the catheter, disconnection of the antibacterial filter and leakage of solution through the skin puncture site. These problems can result in the early loss of up to one in five epidurals, so catheters need to be firmly secured and held in place by a suitable fixative device.

REFERENCES

Arendt-Nielsen, L. and Bjerring, P. (1988) Laser-induced pain for evaluation of local analgesia: a comparison of topical application (EMLA) and local injection (Lidocaine). *Anaesthesia and Analgesia*, **67**, 115–23.

Arrowsmith, J. and Campbell, C. (2000) A comparison of local anaesthetics for venepunture. *Archives of Diseases in Childhood: Fetal and Neonatal Edition*, **82** (4), 309–10.

Berde, C. (1994) Epidural analgesia in children. *Canadian Journal of Anaesthesia*, **41**, 555–60.

Bhat, R., Chari, G., Gulati, A. *et al.* (1990) Pharmaco-kinetics of a single dose of morphine in pre-term infants during the first week of life. *Journal of Paediatrics*, **117**, 477–81.

Bosenberg, A. (1995) Skin epidural distance in children. *Anaesthesia*, **50**, 895–7.

Bray, R., Woodhams, A., Vallis, C. *et al.* (1996) A double-blind comparison of morphine infusion and patient controlled analgesia in children. *Paediatric Anaesthesia*, **6**, 121–7.

Cheung, S., Booker, P., Franks, R. and Pozzi, M. (1997) Serum concentrations of bupivacaine during prolonged continuous para-vertebral infusion in young infants. *British Journal of Anaesthesia*, **79**, 9–13.

Craig, K. (1992) The facial expression of pain: better than a thousand words? *American Pain Society Journal*, **1**, 153–62.

Dahl, J., Rosenberg, J., Hansen, B. *et al.* (1992) Differential analgesic effects of low-dose epidural morphine and morphine-bupivacaine at rest and during mobilisation after major abdominal surgery. *Anesthesia & Analgesia*, **74**, 362–5.

Dunnett, S. (1996) A study to compare the speed of onset, degree and duration of anaestheia produced by Ametop Gel, Emla cream and placebo gel in negroid skin type. In: Wolfsen, A. and McCafferty, D. (eds). *Amethocaine Gel A New Development in Effective Percutaneous Local Anaesthesia.* London: RSM Press, pages 52–9.

Dunwoody, J., Reichert, C. and Brown, K. (1997) Compartment syndrome associated with bupivacaine and fentanyl epidural. *Journal of Paediatric Orthopaedics*, **17**, 285–8.

Eyres, R. (1995) Local anaesthetic agents in infancy. *Paediatric Anaesthesia*, **5**, 213–18.

Giaufre, E., Dalens, B. and Gombert, A. (1996) Epidemiology and morbidity of regional anesthesia in children: a one-year prospective survey of the French-Language Society of Paediatric Anaesthesiologists. *Anesthesia & Analgesia*, **83**, 904–12.

Grundy, R., Howard, R. and Evans, J. (1993) Practical management of pain in sickling disorders. *Archives of Diseases in Childhood*, **69**, 256–9.

Hartley, R. and Levene, M. (1995) Opioid pharmacology in the newborn. In: Aynsley Green, A., Ward Platt, M. and Lloyd-Thomas, A. (eds). *Clinical Paediatrics: Stress and Pain in Infancy and Childhood.* London: Baillière, pages 467–93.

Hassan, M., Howard, R. and Lloyd-Thomas, A. (1994) Depth of epidural space in children. *Anasethesia*, **66**, 1085–6.

Henneberg, S., Hole, P., Masden de Haas, I. and Jensen, P. (1993) Epidural morphine for post-operative pain relief in children. *Acta Anaesthesiolgy Scandinavia*, **37**, 664–7.

Hester, N. (1995) Assessment of acute pain. In: Aynsley-Green, A., Ward Platt, M. and Lloyd-Thomas, A. (eds). *Clinical Paediatrics: Stress and Pain in Infancy and Childhood.* London: Baillière Tindall.

Jennings, E. and Fitzgerald, M. (1996) C-fos can be induced in the neonatal rat spinal cord by both noxious and innocuous stimulation. *Pain*, **68**, 301–6.

Kar, S. and Quirion, R. (1995) Neuropeptide receptors in developing an adult rat spinal cord: an in vitro quantitative auto radiography study of calcitonin gene-related peptide, neurokinins, β-opioid, galanin, somatostatin, neurotension and vocative intestinal polypeptide receptors. *Journal of Complete Neurology*, **354**, 253–81.

Kehlet, H. (1994) Postoperative pain relief – what is the issue? *British Journal of Anaesthesia*, **72**, 375–8.

Krechel, S. and Bildner, J. (1995) CRIES: a new neonatal postoperative pain measurement score. Initial testing of validity and reliability. *Paediatric Anaesthesia*, **5**, 53–61.

Larsson, B., Olsson, G. and Lonnqvist, P. (1994) Plasma concentrations of bupivacaine in young infants after continuous epidural infusion. *Paediatric Anaesthesia*, **4**, 159–62.

Lloyd-Thomas, A. and Howard, R. (1994) A pain service for children. *Paediatric Anaesthesia*, **4**, 3–15.

McGrath, P., Johnson, G., Goodman, J. *et al.* (1987) CHEOPS: a behavioral scale for rating postoperative pain in children. In: Fields, H., Dubner, R. and Cervero, F. (eds). *Advances in Pain Research and Therapy.* New York: Raven Press.

McHale, J. and O'Donovan, F. (1997) Post-dural puncture symptoms in a child. *Anaesthesia*, **52**, 688–90.

McNeely, J. and Trentadue, N. (1997) Comparison of patient-controlled analgesia with and without night time morphine infusion following lower extremity surgery in children. *Journal of Pain and Symptom Management*, **13**, 268–73.

McRorie, T., Lynn, A., Nespeca, M. *et al.* (1992) The maturation of morphine clearance and metabolism. *American Journal of Diseases in Childhood*, **146**, 972–6.

Maxwell, L. Martin, L. and Yaster, M. (1994) Bupivacaine-induced cardiac toxicity in neonates: successful treatment with intravenous phonation. *Anaesthesiology*, **80**, 682–6.

Meunier, J., Norwood, P., Dartayet, B. *et al.* (1997) Skin abscess with lumbar epidural catheterisation in infants: is it dangerous? Report of two cases. *Anesthesia & Analgesia*, **84**, 1248–9.

Peutrell, J., Holder, K. and Gregory, M. (1997) Plasma bupivacaine concentrations associated with continuous extra-dural infusion in babies. *British Journal of Anaesthesia*, **78**, 160–2.

Peutrell, J. and Hughes, D. (1995) A grand-mal convulsion in a child in association with a continuous epidural infusion of bupivacaine. *Anaesthesia*, **50**, 563–4.

Royal College of Anaesthetists (2001) *Bulletin 8 – Guidance on the Provision of Paediatric Anaesthetic Services*. London: Royal College of Anaesthetists.

Southall, D. (1997) Over-dosage of opiate from patient controlled analgesia devices. *British Medical Journal*, **309**, 1002.

Sparshott, M. (1996) The development of a clinical distress scale for ventilated newborn infants: identification of pain and distress based on validated behavioural scores. *Journal of Neonatal Nursing*, April 5–11.

Tyler, D., Tu, A., Douthit, J. and Chapman, C. (1993) Toward validation of pain measurement tools for children: a pilot study. *Pain*, **52**, 301–9.

Ved, S., Pinosky, M. and Nicodemus, H. (1993) Ventricular tachycardia and brief cardiovascular collapse in two infants after caudal anaesthesia using bupivacaine epinephrine solution. *Anaesthesiology*, **79**, 1121–3.

Wilson, P. and Lloyd-Thomas, A. (1993) An audit of extra-dural infusion analgesia in children using bupivacaine and diamorphine, *Anasthesia*, **48**, 718–23.

Wong, D., Hockenberry-Eaton, M., Wilson, D. *et al.* (2001) *Wong's Essentials of Pediatric Nursing*. St Louis: Mosby,

Wood, C., Goresky, G., Klassen, K. *et al.* (1994) Complications of continuous epidural infusions for postoperative analgesia in children. *Canadian Journal of Anesthesia*, **41**, 613–20.

Woolf, C. (1994) The dorsal horn: state dependent sensory processing and the generation of pain. In: Wall, P. and Melzack, R. (eds). *The Textbook of Pain*. London: Churchill Livingstone, pages 101–12.

Yu, D. and Barr, G. (1995) The induction of fos-like immuno-reactivity by noxious thermal, mechanical and chemical stimuli in the lumbar spinal cord of infant rats. *Pain*, **60**, 257–65.

8

Patient Observations

CAROLYN MIDDLETON

Clinical Nurse Specialist in Pain Management, Nevill Hall Hospital,
Abergavenny, South Wales

Close monitoring of patients receiving continuous epidural analgesia is an essential part of the role of the nurse working in an acute surgical area. This chapter will give an overview of the nature and frequency of the observations required although local policy should also be consulted.

MONITORING OF A PATIENT PRIOR TO LEAVING RECOVERY

Prior to leaving the recovery room the patient with an epidural infusion who has also undergone a general anaesthetic should be conscious with return of reflexes and should be able to maintain his or her own airway. Respiratory rate and pattern should be adequate, with no concerns regarding central and peripheral perfusion. Blood pressure, pulse and oxygen saturations should have returned to preoperative levels and be stable. Adequate analgesia should have been achieved via the epidural and attention should be directed to the effects of any residual motor blockade following regional anaesthesia.

The recovery staff should hand over their patient to the ward or escort nurse with all relevant documentation. The patient should then be transported back to the ward area, accompanied by a qualified nurse with oxygen, suction and monitoring equipment as appropriate to the patient's condition.

Epidural Analgesia in Acute Pain Management. Edited by Carolyn Middleton.
© 2006 by John Wiley & Sons, Ltd. ISBN 0-470-01964-6

MONITORING OF A PATIENT IN A SURGICAL WARD

The Royal College of Anaesthetists (RCA) and the Association of Anaesthetists of Great Britain and Ireland (AAGBI) (2004) have made several specific recommendations regarding the ward areas where an epidural service is available. These include the following.

* Wards or units where the technique of continuous epidural infusion is employed frequently enough to ensure expertise and safety.
* Patients receiving continuous epidural analgesia should be nursed only in individual rooms that are close to the nurses' station.
* Patients receiving continuous epidural analgesia must always be under the direct supervision of a nurse, or nurses, trained in the management of continuous epidural analgesia and able to be with the patient within seconds of being summoned.
* There must be 24 hour access to anaesthetic advice for the management of continuous epidural analgesia. For many hospitals a resident anaesthetist will provide this advice.
* There must be 24 hour availability of staff trained to recognise and manage the more serious complications of continuous epidural analgesia.
* There must be 24 hour availability of a resuscitation team with a resident doctor who is competent in resuscitation.
* A system of communication should exist to inform the anaesthetists of inadequate ward staffing if continuous epidural analgesia is planned for a patient from that ward.

FREQUENCY OF OBSERVATIONS

Monitoring should take place throughout the entire period of continuous epidural analgesia, however patients' observations should be recorded most frequently in the first 6 to 12 hours after the epidural infusion has been established. Observations should also be performed more frequently following a top-up bolus or after any change has been made to infusion rates.

Initially, after insertion of the catheter observations should be recorded every 15 minutes for the first two hours, hourly for the next four hours and two hourly thereafter unless there is cause for concern. After the first 24 hours the patient's normal sleep pattern (22.00–06.00 hours) should be disrupted as little as possible but routine manual pulse, respiratory rate and sedation scores along with infusion device recordings should continue two hourly.

TYPE OF OBSERVATIONS

Respiratory Rate

Normal regulation of breathing is a complex process that relies on both peripheral and central control. Respiration is regulated by a variety of factors including the chemoreceptor response to low arterial partial pressure of oxygen (low PaO_2) or to an increase in arterial partial pressure of carbon dioxide (high $PaCO_2$) by raising the rate and/or the depth of respiration. Opioids can have the effect of reducing respiratory stimulation by significant depression of the CO_2 response but slight increases in $PaCO_2$. Acute pain stimulates respiration and helps to antagonise the respiratory depressant effects of opioids (Borgbjerg *et al.*, 1996).

Respiratory depression is relatively uncommon, although a much feared complication of opioid administration. Respiratory rate is therefore used as a key indicator of clinical respiratory depression. When respiratory rate is counted it should be the unstimulated rate, i.e. before the patient is roused. It is generally accepted that a rate of less than eight breaths per minute indicates respiratory depression, however it is useful to record baseline respiratory rate for each patient prior to commencement of epidural infusion.

Depression of level of consciousness can also be used as a useful guide to observing clinical effect in patients receiving opioids as respiratory depression is almost always preceded by a reduced conscious state.

Sedation Scoring

According to McCaffery and Pasero (2002) no patient has succumbed to opioid induced respiratory depression while being awake; this is because less opioid is required to produce sedation than respiratory depression. Therefore, if patients usually show signs of sedation before they show signs of respiratory depression sedation scoring can be used as a sensitive indicator of the likelihood of respiratory depression. An example of a sedation scoring tool that can be used in clinical practice is:

0 = fully awake
1 = drowsy but easy to rouse
2 = mostly sleeping but rousable
3 = difficult to rouse.

The numerical value that represents the sedation score of the patient should be recorded on the patient observation chart so that trends of decreasing sedation can easily be detected.

Oxygen Saturations

Oxygen therapy is commonly used postoperatively where there is evidence or a likelihood of deficiency in the normal oxygen delivery pathway. Oxygen is usually delivered via a facemask with a flow regulator, the majority of oxygen delivered via such devices is given at a rate to maintain an oxygen saturation level above 95% and prevent hypoxia (Anderson, 2003). Saturations refer to haemoglobin that has four binding sites to which the oxygen molecules can attach creating oxyhaemoglobin which the pulse oximeter measures (Clancy and McVicar, 2002).

Supply of oxygen to tissues and organs is crucial and is dependent on cardiac output, haemoglobin and oxygen saturations. When the demand for oxygen is not being satisfied, cell injury results. Monitoring of oxygen saturations via pulse oximetry has become a routine procedure for postsurgical patients in a bid to help identify early change in physiological parameters (Howell, 2002).

There are several factors that can contribute to poor signals from the pulse oximeter leading to inaccurate readings, these are:

- reduced tissue perfusion;
- poor peripheral circulation;
- hypothermia;
- strong light;
- hypovolaemia;
- pulmonary or cardiac disease.

Therefore, pulse oximetry readings should be treated with caution and should only be used in conjunction with respiratory assessment including rate, rhythm and depth of respiration (Casey, 2001).

Blood Pressure

Blood pressure is the force exerted by blood on the vessel walls; it is dependent on the heart's pumping force, blood volume, elasticity of the arteries and resistance to flow. Blood pressure is essential to ensure adequate blood flow including oxygenation of tissues, cells and vital organs (Trim, 2004). The systolic blood pressure is the pressure that occurs in the major arteries after ventricular contraction and gives an indication of the integrity of the heart, arteries and arterioles. The diastolic blood pressure gives an indication of blood vessel resistance. With vasoconstriction the diastolic pressure will be elevated and with vasodilation it will fall.

Epidural blockade can cause hypotension as local anaesthetics can cause a degree of vasodilation, however, staff must be aware that the most likely cause of postoperative hypotension is surgical bleeding causing hypovolaemia (RCA and AAGBI, 2004).

Having a baseline blood pressure reading recorded prior to commencement of epidural infusion can be a useful guide postoperatively of any deterioration.

Temperature

Temperature represents the balance between heat gain and loss. The normal core body temperature is between 36 and 37°C, which needs to be maintained in order for cellular metabolic activity to take place (Trim, 2005a). Control of temperature is regulated by the hypothalamus and core body temperature measurements are taken to assess any deviation from the normal range. Extreme rises in temperature, known as pyrexia, can occur and may be caused by a variety of reasons including infection or more severely sepsis.

As infection in the epidural space can lead to catastrophic outcomes (Chapter 10), it is important to monitor temperature in patients receiving epidural analgesia and identify any pyrexia as it may be an indicator of potential infection.

Pulse

The heart's pumping action causes the arterial walls to expand and contract; this can be monitored manually in a number of places where arteries lie close to the skin surface, i.e. the radial or ulna, carotid or femoral arteries. The pulse is a wave-like sensation indicative of arteries expanding during the systolic phase and recoiling during the diastolic phase of each cardiac cycle. Therefore, assessment of the pulse provides an insight into the cardiovascular function of the patient (Trim, 2005b).

A resting pulse should be between 60 and 100 beats per minute (80–140 in babies up to two years old, and 75–120 in children aged 2–6 years old). Tachycardia is characterised by an adult pulse rate of greater than 100 beats per minute (Trim, 2004). Causes of tachycardia include pyrexia, stress, heart disease, infection or hypovolaemia due to either blood loss or vasodilation; here the blood pressure usually drops with a compensatory increase in pulse to maintain cardiac output. Local anaesthetic drugs are known to cause vasodilation, however, before attributing an increased pulse rate to the epidural, a thorough check should be made for any signs of bleeding attributed to the surgical operation.

As the stress response can cause a rise in pulse rate appropriate pain assessment should be carried out to establish the efficacy of the epidural.

Pain Assessment

Pain is one of the most complex human experiences and nurses have a moral, ethical, humanitarian and professional responsibility to provide an adequate standard of pain assessment and documentation (Dimond, 2002). Amount of tissue damage is not an accurate predictor of intensity or existence of pain and a validated pain assessment tool should be used and the scores or information obtained should be documented as the fifth vital sign (American Pain Society, 1995). A major stumbling block to achieving effective acute pain management is the absence of (or inaccurate) assessment of the patient's pain.

There are numerous clinical tools currently available to measure pain intensity, they were originally designed for research, but have since been adapted for use in the clinical arena. Although they vary in content, structure and complexity the main aims of the pain assessment tool are:

- to enhance the patient's self-report of pain;
- to determine the intensity, quality and duration of pain;
- to aid diagnosis;
- to determine the most appropriate method of providing pain relief;
- to evaluate the efficacy of treatment;
- to avoid judgement bias of healthcare professionals;
- to ensure a structured, documented approach to pain management.

One-dimensional Tools

One-dimensional tools are simple and quick to use and understand. They are considered accurate measures of pain intensity providing the pain is assessed on movement.

Three potential types of pain measurement are:

1. verbal rating scale (verbal descriptor scale or categorical scale);
2. numerical rating scale;
3. visual analogue scale.

The disadvantages of one-dimensional tools are that they oversimplify the pain experience and some patients find it difficult to express their subjective multidimensional experience of pain as a number or a mark on a line.

Verbal Rating Scales

A verbal rating scale (VRS) consists of a list of words used to describe pain. The number of words used varies and up to 20 different VRSs have been developed. The words are usually listed in order from the least to the most intense pain. The words are sometimes assigned a score to represent the level of pain, for example 0 = no pain, 1 = mild pain, 2 = moderate pain and 3 = severe pain. Patients arc asked to use the word that best describes their experience of pain and the corresponding number is recorded on the patient's observational monitoring chart.

The advantages of verbal rating scales are that:

- they enable patients to express their pain in words rather than in numbers allowing them to describe their pain;
- patients find them easy to understand and use;
- they can be quick and easy to teach to patients;
- they are easy to score and to document.

This type of scale is useful in the postoperative situation and also for patients with limited literacy skills. These scales can be easily translated into different languages, although care needs to be taken that the translation is accurate (Davidhizar and Giger, 2004).

The main disadvantage of a VRS is that the different words used to describe pain have different meanings for different people. Therefore, patients may be unable to find a word that accurately reflects their experience of pain from the limited choice.

Numerical Rating Scales

Numerical rating scales (NRSs) and verbal numerical scales consist of a set of numbers, usually 0–10, represented along a horizontal line and may be represented as a pain thermometer or a box scale. There is sometimes an anchor word at each end of the line, for example at 0 = no pain and at 10 = worst pain imaginable. Patients are asked to point or draw around the number that best describes their pain intensity. Alternatively, patients can verbalise the number that best represents their pain score.

This type of scale is quick and easy to use and understand. It also has several practical advantages, for example it is extremely easy to teach, score and document and can be either written or verbal. An adaptation of the numerical rating scale is available in different languages from the Pain Society website at www.painsociety.org/pain_scales.html.

Visual Analogue Scales

A visual analogue scale (VAS) consists of a 10 cm horizontal line with no words or numbers along its length, there are usually word anchors at each end point such as no pain and worst pain imaginable. The patient is asked to mark on the line in pen or pencil between the two end points the place that best reflects their current pain intensity.

The advantages of this type of scale are that it is relatively easy to teach, understand and score. It is quick to use, although some patients may find it confusing. It can be quite difficult to document and some patients find it difficult immediately postoperatively to use a pencil to mark the line in the place that represents their pain intensity. The VAS is more complicated than the NRS and requires greater cognitive skills (Rowbotham and Macintyre, 2003).

Multidimensional Tools

Multidimensional pain assessment tools are more useful in the assessment of chronic pain than of acute pain. They are often complex, lengthy to complete, include a series of questions about pain and quality of life and frequently include a body map.

In order to gain full co-operation and understanding from the patient it is useful to show the patient the tool prior to their surgery. The pain measurement tool can be invaluable in helping patients to communicate their subjective experience of pain which cannot then be misinterpreted or underestimated by health professionals; this type of self-report is regarded as the gold standard of pain measurement.

Pain should be assessed and reassessed frequently during the immediate postoperative period (and after any intervention such as an epidural bolus top-up) to monitor efficacy of the treatment. The frequency of pain assessment should be altered to correspond with the patient's condition and the assessment should always be made on movement rather than at rest. If a score obtained shows an unacceptable level of pain, prompt action should be taken to relieve it, ensuring that patient safety is paramount (Chapter 10).

In addition to performing routine postoperative observations, observations specific to epidural analgesia should be performed and recorded.

Checking the Dermatomal Level of Block

Nurses caring for patients should be aware of the expected level of dermatomal block and be able to check if the height of the block is increasing or decreasing. As the nociceptive fibres (A delta and C fibres) carry information relating to temperature as well as pain, it is possible to determine the level of the block using ice or ethyl chloride. The ice should be put on the patient's skin and he or she should be asked to identify when there is a change in temperature sensation. Ice put on unblocked dermatomal skin areas will feel the full coldness; on partially blocked areas the ice will feel slightly cold; and on well blocked areas touch only of the ice cube will be felt and there will be no cold sensation noted. Checking of block level should take place every eight hours or more frequently if there is any doubt about an adequate block being maintained.

It is helpful if the required level of block (which relates directly to the surgical incision site) is documented by the anaesthetist at the time of surgery, e.g. desired level of block – upper T4 and lower T12 for a midline abdominal wound. A dedicated monitoring chart which incorporates such information is a useful way of conveying this information from the anaesthetist to all health professionals who are involved in the care of the patient postoperatively.

Monitoring is essential so that potentially serious complications can be detected early. An increasing degree of motor weakness implies excessive epidural drug administration, dural penetration of the catheter or the development of either an epidural haematoma or an abscess.

If development of an epidural abscess is suspected then an urgent MRI scan is required to confirm (or otherwise) the presence of the abscess. If nerve root or spinal compression is diagnosed immediate surgical decompression is required (Chapter 10).

Fluid Balance

Sympathetic blockade from the local anaesthetic drug, pre-existing dehydration and interoperative fluid loss in the postoperative patient may require large fluid volumes as replacement. Also urinary retention may occur if the patient is not catheterised.

Checking of Epidural Insertion Site

The insertion site should be regularly checked for any signs of infection. This inspection should take place at least once per shift while the catheter is in place. It should be possible to view the entry site through the transparent dressing, which should not be removed for inspection. After removal of the epidural catheter the site should be checked once per day for 48 hours.

Redness, swelling or purulent discharge at the entry site will necessitate removal of the epidural catheter as soon as possible. The site should be swabbed and the tip of the catheter sent to the bacteriology laboratory for culture and sensitivity (C and S) examination. Identification of sepsis will necessitate discussion with the microbiology department and possible antibiotic therapy. Possible local infection should also be suspected in a patient who complains of increasing back pain or tenderness at the epidural catheter entry site, or in the patient who has an unexplained raised temperature.

Prevention of infection is paramount and strict aseptic technique must be employed when dealing with a patient with an epidural catheter in place. The use of an in-line filter and maintenance of a closed system will help to reduce risks (Chapter 3). A catheter that becomes inadvertently disconnected should not be reconnected. The infusion should be discontinued and the catheter removed in order to prevent the risk of introducing infection into the epidural space. In this case an alternative analgesic technique will need to be employed.

Inspection of the epidural site also involves checking for leaking of epidural solution. If a small amount of leaking is evident but the patient is well analgesed the epidural can continue to run. However, the practitioner should be aware that fluid around the epidural site increases the potential risk of infection.

If there is a significant leaking of epidural fluid from the catheter site it is likely that the catheter is no longer located in the epidural space. In such cases the analgesia is not likely to be achieved and removal of the epidural and commencement of an appropriate alternative analgesic technique may be required.

The dressing covering the epidural catheter should not routinely be removed although guidance should be taken from the dressing manufacturer's instructions for use along with local policy. The purpose of this dressing is to help anchor the epidural catheter, to maintain asepsis and to minimise the risk of infection. The dressing should be occlusive to enable observation of the site without disturbing it.

If it is necessary to remove the dressing at any time the procedure should be explained to the patient. A trolley should be prepared with a sterile field to provide an aseptic working surface. The patient should be positioned comfortably on their side or sitting forward so that the site is easily accessible. The old dressing should be removed and placed in a disposable bag. Hands should be washed with an appropriate bactericidal hand rub. The entry site should be cleaned with sodium chloride 0.9% solution. It is necessary to ensure the catheter is well secured to the skin and a transparent occlusive dressing should be applied over the whole area. Hands should be re-washed with bactericidal soap and water after completing the procedure.

Checking of Patent Intravenous Access

Patent intravenous access is essential because if the patient's respiratory function declines it may be necessary to administer the opioid antagonist naloxone. Intravenous administration provides the most rapid onset of action.

Checking the Epidural Device

Staff must only use epidural devices if they have been appropriately trained, as they are accountable for their actions or omissions (Chapter 11) (Nursing and Midwifery Council, 2004).

The epidural infusion device readings should be recorded every two hours and should include rate of infusion and the total volume of epidural solution infused. Two qualified staff must verify the epidural infusion device programme and the drug label against the prescription at the commencement of the infusion after every shift change and after any alteration to the infusion. This information should be documented accordingly on the dedicated patient monitoring chart.

Infusion Rate

If a continuous only delivery system is used it may be necessary for the registered nurse to adjust the rate of the epidural infusion within the prescribed limits. The infusion rate should be influenced by the patient's age and general condition, by the level of insertion of the epidural catheter in relation to the dermatomal area that requires blocking and by the cocktail of drugs being delivered (Chapter 4). The combination of an opioid with a local anaesthetic is thought to allow lower rates of infusion than using either drug in isolation.

If a patient is experiencing pain it may be necessary to increase the rate of the infusion (within the prescribed limits). If the patient has a marked motor block it may be appropriate to decrease the rate (Chapter 10).

ORTHOPAEDIC SURGERY

Masking of compartment syndrome by extradural blockade has been a long-standing concern in both orthopaedic and vascular surgery (Dunwoody *et al.*, 1997). For this reason an epidural infusion may not be the most suitable mode of delivery of analgesic drugs to patients at high risk of developing a compartment syndrome (RCA and AAGBI, 2004).

Pain is one of the predominant warning signs for compartment syndrome, therefore complete eradication of pain through the use of epidural infusion may mask increasing compartmental pressures. Also if there is a degree of altered sensation caused by the local anaesthetic, this may mask any paraesthesia caused by ischaemic nerves within the affected compartment. Rimmer (2002) has also suggested that the vasodilating effects of the local anaesthetic from epidural infusions may actually increase the risk of compartment syndrome by adding to the increase of pressure within a defined lower limb compartment. Therefore, if epidurals are utilised extra vigilance must be taken when observing orthopaedic and vascular patients.

POLICY DOCUMENTS

Local trust policy documents used to guide the epidural service should give clear guidance to staff regarding the type and frequency of observations required for patients receiving an epidural infusion. This guidance should also outline the appropriate action to be taken if the patient's observations significantly digress from pre-epidural standard values of each patient. Potentially serious problems can usually be averted if detected early and acted upon (Chapter 10).

DOCUMENTATION

Contemporaneous records must be kept of events throughout the period that the epidural infusion is in use. The records should reflect: the discussion regarding the obtaining of consent prior to catheter insertion (see Chapters 1 and 2); the insertion technique itself, i.e. position of the patient; evidence of obtaining loss of resistance and therefore identification of the epidural space; the length of catheter from the skin to the epidural space and the length left within the epidural space (Chapter 3); and the prescription for the epidural infusion including in the case of PCEA bolus dose size, lockout time and background continuous infusion rates (Chapter 5). The patient records must also provide evidence of frequent and appropriate monitoring of all aspects of the patient's condition including inspection of the epidural insertion site. Details of the infusion device checks should be documented along with notes relating to any complications or adverse event that may have occurred.

Details of the prescription for the epidural infusion, the provision of intravenous fluids, oxygen therapy, the opioid antagonist naloxone and balanced analgesia can be preprinted on the patient's prescription chart or dedicated observation chart.

REFERENCES

American Pain Society (1995) Pain: the fifth vital sign. Available at: www.ampainsoc/advacacy/fifth.htm (accessed 2/6/05).

Anderson, I. (2003) *Care of the Critically Ill Surgical Patient*, 2nd edn. London: Arnold.

Borgbjerg, F., Nielsen, K. and Franks, J. (1996) Experimental pain stimulates respiration and attenuates morphine-induced respiratory depression: a controlled study in human volunteers. *Pain*, **64**, 123–8.

Casey, G. (2001) Oxygen transport and the use of pulse oximetry. *Nursing Standard*, **15** (47), 46–53.

Clancy, J. and McVicar, A. (2002) *Physiology and Anatomy: a Homeostatic Approach*, 2nd edn. London: Arnold.

Davidhizar, R. and Giger, J. (2004) A review of the literature on care of clients in pain who are culturally diverse. *International Nursing Reviews*, **51**, 47–55.

Dimond, B. (2002) *Legal Aspects of Pain Management*. Salisbury: Quay Books.

Dunwoody, J., Reichert, C. and Brown, K. (1997) Compartment syndrome associated with bupivacaine and fentanyl epidural. *Journal of Paediatric Orthopaedics*, **17**, 285–8.

Howell, M. (2002) Pulse oximetry: an audit of nursing and medical staff understanding. *British Journal of Nursing*, **11** (3), 191–7.

McCaffery, M. and Pasero, C. (2002) Monitoring sedation. *American Journal of Nursing*, **102** (2), 67–8.

Nursing and Midwifery Council (2004) *Code of Professional Conduct, Standards for Conduct, Performance and Ethics*. London: NMC.

Rimmer, J. (2002) Appropriate pain management in orthopaedic trauma care. *Journal of Bone and Joint Surgery (American)*, **84A** (8), 1479–80.

Rowbotham, D. and Macintyre, P. (2003) *Clinical Pain Management: Acute Pain*. London: Arnold.

Royal College of Anaesthetists and Association of Anaesthetists of Great Britain and Ireland (2004) *Epidurals for Pain Relief after Surgery*. London: RCA/AAGBI.

Trim, J. (2004) Performing a comprehensive physiological assessment. *Nursing Times*, **100** (50), 38–42.

Trim, J. (2005a) Monitoring temperature. *Nursing Times*, **101** (20), 30–1.

Trim, J. (2005b) Monitoring pulse. *Nursing Times*, **101** (21), 30–1.

9

Discontinuation and Removal of the Epidural Catheter

CAROLYN MIDDLETON

Clinical Nurse Specialist in Pain Management, Nevill Hall Hospital, Abergavenny, South Wales

Epidural infusions should be used for a maximum of seven days and then the catheter must be removed as the risk of infection increases exponentially. This chapter aims to give an overview of the issues that should be considered prior to removing an epidural catheter, including the patient's wishes, the availability of alternative routes for administration of analgesic drugs, efficacy of the epidural and anticoagulant therapy. The chapter will also provide the clinician with a detailed account of the procedure required for removing an epidural catheter and the follow-up care necessary for the forthcoming 48 hours.

LENGTH OF DURATION OF EPIDURAL INFUSION

The length of time for which patients require epidural analgesia varies; it is dependent on the type of surgery performed, the patients' condition and their response to pain. Technical problems with the epidural catheter including leakage at the site of entry, catheter occlusion, catheter disconnection and inadvertent falling out of the catheter result in premature discontinuation of epidural analgesia in 11–17% of cases (Rowney and Doyle, 1998). Where the epidural infusion is trouble free the average duration of an infusion is between

Epidural Analgesia in Acute Pain Management. Edited by Carolyn Middleton.
© 2006 by John Wiley & Sons, Ltd. ISBN 0-470-01964-6

48 and 72 hours for orthopaedic joint surgery and often up to five days for general abdominal or thoracic surgery (Murdock, 2005). Epidural catheters cannot remain in place after seven days as the risk of infection rises exponentially with every day that passes.

PRIOR TO REMOVING THE EPIDURAL CATHETER

Prior to removal of the epidural there are several issues that require consideration. Firstly, the severity of pain and the epidural infusion rate. If the epidural is working well and controlling the pain and it has not been in place for more than five days it may be appropriate to reduce the infusion rate prior to removal. This will enable the clinician to assess the patient's response to the reduced analgesia. Regular pain assessment must continue and providing the patient remains comfortable after 3–4 hours the epidural can be removed. If the patient has a significant increase in pain the infusion rate should be adjusted to the previous level and the epidural continued.

Epidural analgesia should only be discontinued when the patient's pain can be effectively managed by other means, or if the patient is experiencing unacceptable complications or adverse effects as a consequence of the epidural analgesia (Chapter 10).

If the patient has severe pain despite the epidural being in place and every effort has been made to adjust the epidural (Chapter 10), then it is probably appropriate to abandon the epidural infusion and provide the patient with alternative analgesia.

The second consideration is to determine which routes are available for alternative administration of analgesia. If the patient is unable to tolerate any oral fluids an intravenous patient controlled device (IV PCA) is probably the most appropriate. If IV PCA is considered, an evaluation of the patient's mental capacity and physical dexterity to manipulate the demand button should be made, if either is problematic, PCA would not be appropriate.

The majority of patients convert to oral analgesia on cessation of epidural pain relief, therefore the epidural infusion should continue until the patient is able to tolerate a minimum of 60 ml of fluid each hour so that the gut is capable of absorbing the oral medication.

The patient's wishes must also be considered during the decision-making process. He or she should be involved in discussions and given sufficient information about alternative analgesic agents for an informed decision to be made.

When a decision is made to stop the epidural, the substitute analgesia should be started at an appropriate time. Intravenous alternatives should not be started until the epidural has been stopped as IV administration has a rapid onset of action time. Opioids given by the IV route would increase the possibility of adverse effects being experienced, particularly respiratory depression.

If oral medication is chosen, the first dose should be administered approximately 30 minutes before stopping the epidural infusion. This will allow time for the pain killer to be absorbed through the lining of the gut before the effects of the epidural infusion recede.

ANTICOAGULANT THERAPY CONSIDERATIONS

Any patient receiving anticoagulation or thromboprophylaxis is at greater risk of haematoma; therefore it is essential to consider anticoagulant therapy prior to removal of the epidural catheter (Cox, 2002; British National Formulary, 2004). A safe period of time must elapse between the administration of an anticoagulant and catheter removal in order to avoid the formation of an epidural haematoma.

Minihep

Minihep (low dose standard heparin)

* Epidural catheter cannot be removed until 4 hours after the last minihep injection.
* Do not give the next minihep injection until 4 hours have elapsed since removal of the epidural catheter.

Low Molecular Weight Heparin, e.g. Enoxaparin/Tinzaparin

Partial anticoagulation with low molecular weight heparin (LMWH)

* Epidural catheter cannot be removed until 12 hours after the last injection.
* Do not give next low molecular weight heparin until 4 hours have elapsed since removal of the epidural catheter.

Arixtra (Fondaparinux Sodium)

* Epidural catheter cannot be removed until 36 hours after the last injection.
* Do not give next dose of Arixtra until 12 hours have elapsed since removal of the epidural catheter.

NSAIDs/Aspirin

* NSAIDs/aspirin do not increase the risk of epidural haematoma.
* Catheter removal and dosing with NSAIDs carry no time constrictions.

(Wheatley *et al.*, 2001)

Although it is an absolute contraindication to insert an epidural catheter into a patient with coagulation defects or who is receiving anticoagulation therapy (i.e. warfarin or heparin), occasionally a patient may suffer a thrombotic event postoperatively and be anticoagulated during the period that the epidural infusion is in progress (Horlocker and Wedel, 1998). In such cases a consultant anaesthetist should be involved in the decision to remove the epidural catheter and bloods should be taken to review the clotting status of the patient.

Heparin Infusion

* Stop heparin infusion for 3 hours, check activated partial thromboplastin time (APTT) and contact the anaesthetist with blood results prior to removal.

Warfarin

* Check international normalised ratio (INR) and contact anaesthetist with result prior to removal of the epidural catheter.

An epidural haematoma should be suspected in patients who complain of severe back pain a few hours or days following any central neuraxial block or with any prolonged or abnormal neurological deficit. This may include sensory loss, parasthesia, muscle weakness and disturbance of bladder control and/or anal sphincter tone. If haematoma does occur early orthopaedic or neurosurgical referral for decompression is required. Even with early recognition, the morbidity of this condition is still very high (Chapter 10).

REMOVAL PROCEDURE

Reassure the Patient

Explain fully to the patient exactly what to expect and reassure the patient that the procedure is not at all painful.

Prepare the Trolley

The trolley should be prepared in advance and should include:

* sterile gloves;
* sterile field towel;

- dressing pack;
- wound spray;
- plaster or wound dressing (preferably transparent);
- specimen pot if catheter tip is to be sent for culture and sensitivity (C and S) (not routine);
- sterile scissors if catheter tip is to be sent for C and S.

Positioning of the Patient

The spine needs to be flexed; the patient should be put into (preferably) the same position as they were in when the catheter was inserted (Chapter 3), this information should be documented on the anaesthetic chart. An assistant may be required to support the patient while the procedure is being carried out.

Removal of Epidural Catheter

The epidural catheter should be removed under sterile conditions. Remove the dressing that is covering the epidural catheter. Using gloves and a sterile field to work from, gently apply traction to the catheter; there may be a slight initial resistance but the catheter should then slide out easily. If it does not do so, reposition the patient with the spine further flexed and apply traction again. The catheter should not be made to stretch as there is a slight possibility of the catheter snapping. If the catheter cannot be removed it should be re-secured with a sterile dressing and the anaesthetist called.

Once the catheter has been removed it is important to inspect the tip to ensure that the entire catheter has been removed and that the catheter has not snapped inside the epidural space (Chapman and Day, 2001). Most catheter tips have a coloured marking to denote the tip presence (Figure 9.1). It is important to document in the patient's notes the status of the catheter tip. Although very rare, in the case of the tip shearing off from the rest of the catheter, both the patient and the anaesthetist should be informed. It is unlikely that the tip would be surgically removed. If problems are encountered removing the epidural catheter the anaesthetist and/or acute pain service should be contacted.

If there is any indication that infection may be present, i.e. redness, swelling, discharge from the site, the tip of the catheter should be cut with a pair of sterile scissors, placed into a universal container and sent to the bacteriology laboratory for C and S tests (Murdock, 2005). Any epidural catheter tips that are sent should be followed up by the acute pain service and when the report is available appropriate antibiotic therapy commenced for the patient if indicated. Discussion with the microbiology department may be required.

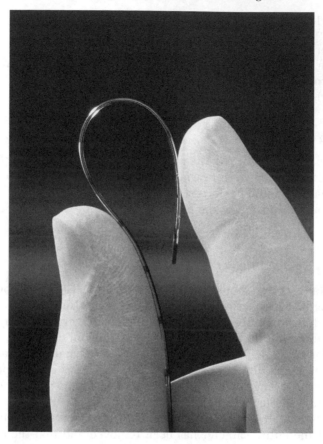

Figure 9.1. Epidural catheter tip. (Reproduced by permission of B-Braun Medical Ltd.)

Re-dressing the Site

Once the catheter has been removed, the site should be cleaned if necessary, dried with a sterile swab and then the site sprayed with a plastic spray and/or a transparent dressing applied for 24 hours.

Observation of the Site

For 48 hours post-removal of the epidural catheter the site should be inspected at least once daily for any signs of infection. If infection is suspected the site can be swabbed and a C and S request made, again it is imperative that results are followed up and acted upon where necessary.

DISPOSAL OF WASTE CONTROLLED DRUGS

The total amount of epidural solution that has been infused should be recorded on the appropriate patient monitoring chart. Any remaining epidural solution (if it contains a controlled drug (CD)) should be disposed of according to local trust policy. It is usual for the details of the drug disposed of to be recorded in the CD register. The entry should include the following information:

- date of disposal;
- amount of drug destroyed;
- name of patient;
- signature of staff involved in disposing of drug, this must be a trained nurse and witnessed by one of the following: nurse, doctor or pharmacist.

FOLLOWING REMOVAL OF THE EPIDURAL CATHETER

PAIN SCORING

Pain scoring should continue after removal of the epidural infusion in order to continue to assess the level of pain that the patient is experiencing (Chapter 8). Pain scoring also allows assessment of efficacy of the new analgesic regimen employed.

BALANCED STEP-DOWN ANALGESIA

It is essential that following discontinuation of the epidural infusion balanced step-down analgesia is employed. This should follow the principles of the World Health Organisation (WHO) analgesic ladder and include a simple analgesic, i.e. paracetamol, an NSAID (where appropriate) and a weak opioid to ensure a synergistic effect (Chapter 4).

REFERENCES

British National Formulary (2004) *BNF 47*. London: British Medical Association and the Royal Pharmaceutical Society of Great Britain.

Chapman, S. and Day, R. (2001) Spinal anatomy and the use of opioids. *Professional Nurse*, **16** (6), 1174–7.

Cox, F. (2002) Making sense of epidural analgesia. *Nursing Times*, **98** (32), 56–8.

Horlocker, T. and Wedel, D. (1998) Spinal and epidural blockade and peri-operative low molecular weight heparin. *Anesthesia & Analgesia*, **8**, 1153–6.

Murdock, J. (2005) Ensuring prompt diagnosis and treatment of epidural abscess. *Nursing Times*, **101** (20), 36–8.

Rowney, D. and Doyle, E. (1998) Epidural and sub-arachnoid blockade in children. *Anaesthesia*, **53** (10), 980–1001.

Wheatley, R., Schug, S. and Watson, D. (2001) Safety and efficacy of postoperative epidural analgesia. *British Journal of Anaesthesia*, **87** (1), 47–61.

10

Troubleshooting

DEE COMERFORD
Clinical Nurse Specialist in Pain Management, Singleton Hospital,
Swansea, South Wales

This chapter is designed not only to answer questions that nurses may have in relation to epidural management, but also to reassure them that epidurals are safe and effective (providing best practice guidelines are in place). Information will be presented relating to the potential problems that may occur with epidural analgesia, the likely incidence of occurrence, how to recognise such problems at an early stage and what steps to take to rectify them.

COMPLICATIONS RELATED TO EPIDURAL INFUSIONS

Although epidurals are generally regarded as a safe and effective means of providing pain management, they are not without risk of complications. Studies such as that of Kurek and Lagares-Garcia (1997) report the overall rate of potentially serious complications at 14%. The adverse effects associated with epidural analgesia are generally related to:

- the epidural needle or catheter;
- inadequate analgesia;
- the opioid and/or local anaesthetic drug;
- the equipment.

Epidural Analgesia in Acute Pain Management. Edited by Carolyn Middleton.
© 2006 by John Wiley & Sons, Ltd. ISBN 0-470-01964-6

Table 10.1. Adverse effects associated with epidural analgesia (Kurek & Largares-Garcia (1997), Macintyre & Ready (2001) and SWPNF (2002 unpublished)

Epidural needle and catheter related:
• Epidural site infection
• Epidural space infection/abscess
• Epidural haematoma
• Inadvertent dural puncture
• Postdural puncture headache
• Epidural catheter migration (intrathecal or systemic)
• Total spinal
• Nerve or spinal cord injury

Inadequate analgesia:
• Related to surgery
• Related to other causes

Opioid and/or local anaesthetic drug related:
• Respiratory depression and sedation
• Hypotension
• Dense and/or high block
• Nausea and vomiting
• Pruritis
• Urinary retention/incontinence
• Hallucination
• Local anaesthetic toxicity

Related to the equipment:
• Leakage from the epidural catheter insertion site
• Disconnection of the epidural catheter from the antibacterial filter
• Epidural catheter dislodgement
• Sheared off epidural catheter tip
• Epidural infusion device

A complete list of adverse effects associated with epidural analgesia is summarised in Table 10.1.

EPIDURAL NEEDLE OR CATHETER RELATED ADVERSE EFFECTS

Major neurological adverse effects are uncommon in patients with epidural analgesia. In a recent study (Giebler *et al.*, 1997) of 4000 patients with thoracic epidurals, the incidence of neurological complications was 3%. Complications included dural puncture, inability to insert the catheter, radicular pain on catheter insertion as well as radicular pain and peripheral nerve palsies after surgery. There were no long-term neurological effects and the study estimated an overall risk of 1 in 1500 (0.07%) for neurological complications, but, this figure may be increased in patients with coagulopathies.

Epidural Site Infection

Epidurals should not be considered for patients with local infection at the site of insertion as this may lead to systemic infection. However, for some patients infection may develop at the epidural site at any time from insertion to removal of the catheter.

In the Burstal *et al.* (1998b) study there was shown to be a highly significant difference in the incidence of site inflammation between a catheter left in situ for three days or less and a catheter left for four days or more; 74% of cases of site inflammation occurred on or after day four. Just over 5% of patients developed catheter site inflammation and, of these, 0.47% of patients required antibiotic therapy for positive cultures of the epidural catheter tips. The authors concluded that the decision to continue with epidural analgesia beyond four days should be made after consideration of a risk–benefit analysis for each individual patient, especially in the presence of localised erythema at the epidural catheter site.

The routine practice of microbiological monitoring of epidural catheter tips is called into question in a study by Steffan *et al.* (2004). Microbiological examination of 502 epidural catheters used for postoperative analgesia, over a five year period, suggested the 29% incidence of positive tip cultures was likely to be caused by contamination on removal of the epidural catheter; no case of spinal epidural infection was observed within six months after epidural catheterisation. It would, therefore, appear to be unnecessary to send catheter tips for microbiological examination unless clinical signs and symptoms dictate it.

However, detection of neurological symptoms such as unusual back tenderness at the site of insertion, pyrexia and raised erythrocyte sedimentation rate (ESR) indicates more than a localised problem and these need to be investigated immediately to rule out epidural abscess formation. Routine monitoring of the epidural site, at least once in every eight hours, is to be advised in order to detect the occurrence of site inflammation and/or infection. Evidence of this needs to be reported to the acute pain service or anaesthetist immediately, as this may warrant early removal of the epidural catheter to prevent further complications.

Epidural Space Infection/Abscess

Infection in the epidural space is an infrequent complication of epidural analgesia (Burstal *et al.*, 1998b). A recent national survey of epidural practices showed an incidence of epidural abscess of approximately 1 in 2000 patients, with associated risk factors including prolonged catheter placement (more than three days) and compromised immune systems (Williams and Wheatley, 2000). However, in recent years there have been an increasing number of reported cases (de Leon-Casasola *et al.*, 1994; Scott *et al.*, 1995).

When it does occur, deep infection is usually due to homogeneous spread but may occur due to direct needling, tracking of superficial infection or solution contamination (Dawson, 1995). Attention to sterile technique, use of sterile pre-prepared solutions, closed dedicated delivery systems and early catheter removal may reduce the risk.

The signs and symptoms of an epidural space infection are similar to those of an epidural haematoma although the onset is slower and may be delayed by days or weeks after the patient has been discharged from hospital (Macintyre and Ready, 2001). Initial presenting symptoms include tenderness at the insertion site, signs of infection and increasing and persistent back pain.

Kindler *et al.* (1998) found that there is a lower incidence of abscess with lumbar epidurals compared with thoracic epidurals. This may be explained by the length of time the epidural remains in place. Thoracic epidurals are generally associated with abdominal surgery and tend to remain in place for longer, whereas lumbar epidurals are more commonly used for orthopaedic surgery and removed after 48–72 hours. Also thoracic catheters are thought to be technically more difficult to insert and therefore there is a greater reluctance to remove them if there is any possibility they may need to be replaced (O'Higgins and Tuckey, 2000).

Monitoring of sensory and motor block is essential for the early detection of this potentially serious complication. An increasing degree of motor weakness may imply the development of cither an epidural abscess or haematoma and requires immediate review by a senior anaesthetist (Wang, 1999). Removal of the epidural catheter is essential and the tip of the catheter must be sent for microbiology, culture and sensitivity tests. If an abscess is suspected, particularly in the presence of neurological deficits, an urgent MRI scan will be required and urgent neurosurgical consultation sought. Surgical decompression within eight hours of the initial onset of neurological signs and symptoms is crucial for a positive patient outcome (Macintyre and Ready, 2001; Justins, 2004).

Epidural Haematoma

Epidural haematoma is a rare but potentially catastrophic adverse effect that may occur in association with epidural analgesia. Risk factors for the development of an epidural haematoma include anticoagulation therapy, difficult needle or catheter insertion and thrombocytopenia (Table 10.2). The risk of epidural haematoma during epidural analgesia is also increased in patients with a history of chronic renal failure (CRF).

Table 10.2. Patients at risk of epidural haematoma (Adapted from Gedney & Lui 1998; Basta & Sloan 1999)

Known coagulopathy
Difficult or traumatic needle or catheter insertion and removal
Thrombocytopenia
Intravenous anticoagulant therapy
Perioperative low molecular weight heparin
Chronic renal failure
Known spinal cord pathology

The mechanism of action is not completely understood (Basta and Sloan, 1999) although the coagulopathy of CRF is thought to be secondary to platelet dysfunction (Aldrete *et al.*, 1971). Antiplatelet therapy and/or aspirin given preoperatively does not increase the risk of haematoma associated with epidural analgesia according to Horlocker *et al.* (1995), although caution is advised. Conversely, combination therapy with heparin and oral anticoagulants has demonstrated an increase in the frequency of spontaneous bleeding at puncture sites and the development of spinal haematomas (Horlocker *et al.*, 2003).

The increasing use of pharmacological prophylaxis for venous thromboembolism has raised concerns that epidural analgesia may be followed by an increased risk of haematoma in the epidural space. The incidence of haematoma after epidural blockade in patients receiving the low molecular weight heparin (LMWH) enoxaparin was estimated at 1 in 2 250 000 in Europe, but 1 in 14 000 in the United States (Scottish Intercollegiate Guidelines Network (SIGN), 2004). The main contributing factor to this variation was the difference in the recommended dose of the LMWH enoxaparin: 40 mg once daily, 12 hours prior to surgery for high risk European patients, compared with 30 mg twice daily, starting one hour after surgery for American patients. Recently, SIGN (2004) has produced recommendations for the prophylaxis of venous thromboembolism in epidural blockade. An example of the recommendations adapted into a guideline for clinical practice can be seen in Table 10.3 (Swansea Acute Pain Management Service, 2004).

A retrospective analysis of case reports has estimated the incidence of epidural haematoma to be 1 in 190 000 (Wulf, 1996). More recently, an extensive review of the literature identified 13 cases of spinal haematoma following 850 000 epidural anaesthetics and, based on this, calculated the incidence to be less than 1 in 150 000 epidurals (Horlocker *et al.*, 2003).

High risk patients need to be monitored closely postoperatively with a neurological review (i.e. assessment of motor and sensory block) at least every four hours in order to detect the early signs of spinal cord compression or ischaemia. New symptoms of severe low back pain and motor and sensory deficits in the lower limbs should alert staff to the possible complication of

Table 10.3. Guidelines for the prophylaxis of venous thromboembolism in epidural blockade (Swansea Acute Pain Management Service – 2004 unpublished)

Coagulation considerations for patients with epidural analgesia

Unfractionated heparin
For patients receiving low dose subcutaneous heparin (5000 IU minihep):
– Insertion or removal of epidural catheter can take place 4 hours before the next dose is due or 4 hours following the last dose administered

Low molecular weight heparins (LMWH)
For patients receiving subcutaneous LMWH (enoxaparin/certoparin):
– LMWH should not be administered 10–12 hours before insertion or removal of epidural catheter
– LMWH can be administered 2 hours post-insertion or removal of an epidural catheter

Epidural Procedure	Timing for the Administration of LMWH
Pre-insertion	≥10–12 hours
Post-insertion	≥2 hours
Pre-removal	≥10–12 hours
Post-removal	≥2 hours

Heparin infusions
For patients receiving intravenous heparin infusions:
– KCCT (kaolin cephalin clotting time) or APTT (activated partial thromboplastin time) should be ≤1.2 times the normal value prior to insertion or removal of epidural catheter
– The heparin infusion should be stopped for 3 hours prior to insertion/removal of epidural catheter and the KCCT or APTT checked.
– The heparin infusion may be restarted 1 hour after insertion/removal of epidural catheter

Warfarin
For patients receiving warfarin:
– International normalised ratio (INR) should be <1.5 prior to insertion or removal of epidural catheter
– Do not start warfarin while an epidural catheter is in situ
– Epidural analgesia is contraindicated for patients who are fully anticoagulated

Antiplatelet agents
Caution is required with patients receiving aspirin, NSAIDs and antiplatelet therapy (clopidogrel, dipyridamole, eptifibatide):
– Review whole clinical picture for sign of bruising/bleeding

Coagulopathy
Consider impact of conditions such as liver failure, pre-eclampsia, thrombocytopenia, etc., on coagulation status:
– if platelets $<100 \times 10^3$ do not proceed
– if in doubt, check coagulation screen and platelet count

epidural haematoma which requires an immediate review by a senior anaesthetist. If epidural haematoma is suspected, MRI and neurosurgical consultation must be undertaken without delay. Importantly, a window of opportunity for surgical decompression of the haematoma is within eight hours of the initial onset of neurological signs and symptoms, to allow the best prospect of a full recovery (Macintyre and Ready, 2001; Horlocker *et al.*, 2003).

Inadvertent Dural Puncture

Dural puncture is an inherent risk during insertion of the epidural catheter because of the close proximity of the epidural and intrathaecal spaces. If the needle or catheter punctures the dura, cerebrospinal fluid (CSF) will be aspirated, requiring the anaesthetist to reinsert the catheter at a different level. Inadvertent dural puncture is not seen as a serious complication, but the patient has an 80% chance of developing a headache (Kingsley, 2001). The overall incidence of dural puncture is reported to be low at 0.16–1.3% although this may be dependent on the experience and skill of the anaesthetist (Rathmell *et al.*, 2003).

CSF–cutaneous fistula is a very rare but potentially serious and life threatening complication of epidural analgesia, and has been reported following accidental dural puncture during epidural insertion. Most cases of fistulae present within 24 hours of epidural catheter removal, but in one case report the fistula presented five days after epidural catheter removal in a postoperative patient, which was subsequently complicated by bacterial meningitis (Abaza and Bogod, 2004). Signs and symptoms of this atypical complication include severe, distressing occipital headache and a 'wet patch' at the epidural site. Unusual features of post dural puncture headache, such as visual and auditory symptoms, may indicate serious neurological complications. Several approaches have been described for the treatment of this rare complication, these include: bed rest in the prone position, prophylactic antibiotics, fluid restriction, figure of eight suture at the skin puncture site, epidural blood patch, lumbar CSF drainage or surgical closure (Abaza and Bogod, 2004).

Post-dural Puncture Headache

If the dura is punctured, by the epidural needle or catheter, a post-dural puncture headache (PDPH) may occur as a result of a loss of CSF through the dural tear. The headache usually begins in the occipital region and radiates to the frontal and orbital regions. The patient may complain of associated cervical muscle spasm. The pain is made worse if the patient sits up or stands and it may be accompanied by nausea, vomiting, sweating, dizziness, stiff neck, tinnitus, photophobia, double vision, inability to focus or seeing spots before the eyes (Kingsley, 2001). In the more severe cases diplopia and other cranial nerve palsies may occur, in very rare cases intracranial bleeding has resulted (Kurek and Lagares-Garcia, 1997).

In one large study (Burstal *et al.*, 1998a) PDPH only occurred in 0.16% of patients. However, the overall incidence of this adverse effect has been reported to range from 16% to 86% (Rathmell *et al.*, 2003).

Treatment consists of bed rest, simple analgesia such as paracetemol +/− codeine on a regular basis and substantial hydration. Caffeine has also proved to be effective. PDPH is usually self-limiting and resolves with this level of intervention in 24–48 hours. However, in some patients the headache persists beyond 72 hours and in these cases an epidural blood patch may be required. The patient's own blood (10–20 ml) is injected into the epidural space, at the level of the dural puncture, where it clots and seals the dural tear. This stops the CSF leak and in 95% of cases the headache resolves.

Epidural Catheter Migration (Intrathecal or Systemic)

The occurrence of epidural catheter migration has long been recognised as a potentially major complication of epidural analgesia. Although it is rare, the catheter has been reported to have migrated into blood vessels, the subdural and subarachnoid spaces (Ravindran *et al.*, 1979; Abouleish and Goldstein, 1986; Phillips *et al.*, 1986). Several studies have looked at the subcutaneous tunnelling of epidural catheters in an attempt to reduce migration, and Bougher *et al.* (1996) showed that this technique prevented only inward catheter migration, with 62% of tunnelled catheters remaining within 0.5 cm of their sited position.

In the recent Burstal *et al.* (1998b) study, catheter migration was detected in 0.32% of patients, with three cases of intravenous catheter migration and one case of subarachnoid migration, which was detected early because of ascending motor block. While an earlier study by Phillips and MacDonald (1987) showed that twice as many epidural catheters migrated inwards as outwards in their obstetric population. They reported one case of subarachnoid injection and one case of intravascular injection, both of which occurred after an inward migration of more than 2 cm. However, other studies (Giebler, 1997; Clark *et al.*, 2001) suggest that a 1 cm inward migration should be considered as significant. Using this as a marker they showed a 13% inward migration rate in their standard group (coiled catheter under a transparent dressing) compared with 4% in the subcutaneous tunnelled group (Burstal *et al.*, 1998b). The more frequently observed problem is that of outward catheter migration and dislodgement from the epidural space (discussed within the equipment related adverse effects section of this chapter).

Total Spinal Blockade

Where catheter migration results in excessive doses of local anaesthetic agents inadvertently being delivered into the intrathecal or spinal space there is the potential to cause total spinal blockade. This can ultimately lead to unconsciousness and cardiovascular collapse. The rostral spread of the local anaesthetic in the CSF pre-empts the occurrence of detrimental effects on the respiratory and cardiovascular systems, owing to the increasing blockade of motor and autonomic nerves (Macintyre and Ready, 2001). Marked sympathetic blockade will lead to severe hypotension and above thoracic level 4 (nipple line) will block the cardio-accelerator fibres to the heart, causing bradycardia. Severe bradycardia and hypotension will require immediate resuscitative measures to prevent the occurrence of cardiac arrest.

A dense motor block of intercostal muscles will reduce a patient's ability to take deep breaths and cough. If the block reaches cervical nerves 3, 4 and 5, which supply the diaphragm, there is a risk of respiratory depression and arrest. Implementation of the epidural scoring scale for arm movements (ESSAM) tool (Table 10.4), as part of the monitoring protocol for patients receiving epidural analgesia, may assist in the early detection and management of this serious complication.

It is vital to treat the early signs and symptoms of a total spinal blockade promptly and effectively to prevent a potentially devastating outcome. Always stop the epidural infusion and summon help urgently. Treatment requires relevant supportive management at each stage, e.g. oxygenation, intubation and ventilation, full cardiac resuscitative measures.

Nerve or Spinal Cord Injury

Neurological complications may occur following placement of the epidural catheter. In a recent study by Giebler (1997) of over 4000 patients receiving thoracic epidural analgesia, 0.2% reported postoperative radicular-type pain which resolved in all cases, once the epidural catheter had been removed.

Persistent spinal nerve root pain and peripheral nerve pain following epidural analgesia have a reported incidence of 0.001–0.6%. Causation is often attributed to retraction or positioning during surgery (Rathmell *et al.*, 2003).

Paraplegia, an extremely rare complication of epidural analgesia, has been reported following epidural haematoma and epidural abscess formation, resulting in compression of the spinal cord (Giebler, 1997). Paraplegia can also result from a decrease in spinal blood flow due to prolonged hypotension, increased intra abdominal pressure, injury to an anterior spinal artery or cross-clamping of the aorta during surgery (Macintyre and Ready, 2001).

Table 10.4. Scoring system based on the ESSAM system (Adapted from Abd Elrazek *et al.* (1999) *Anaesthesia* **54.** Reproduced by permission of the Swansea NHS Trust)

Thoracic Epidurals
Epidural Scoring Scale for Arm Movements – ESSAM Score

- This monitoring and recording scale has been developed to enable easy and safe monitoring of thoracic epidurals. It should help avoid the risk of high cervical blockade, which may affect respiratory function
- Performing the tests:
  1. Handgrip
     Squeeze my fingers (2); do not let me pull them out of your hand
  2. Wrist flexion
     Bend your wrist; do not let me straighten it
  3. Elbow flexion
     Bend your elbow; do not let me straighten it
- Each test is scored on the basis of the absence (–) or presence (+) of muscle power

Grade	Movement			Action
	Hand grip (T1/C8)	Wrist flexion (C7/C8)	Elbow flexion (C5/C6)	
0	+	+	+	Continue same rate, if patient is pain free
1	–	+	+	Reduce rate by 25%, reassure patient
2	–	–	+	Reduce rate by 50%, inform anaesthetist
3	–	–	–	Stop the infusion and call anaesthetist

Monitoring protocols need to be rigorously applied to ensure the early detection and management of potentially devastating neurological adverse effects.

INADEQUATE ANALGESIA

Unrelieved pain may be related to causes other than the surgical procedure or site of injury, therefore a thorough assessment of the patient is necessary to determine the exact nature of the pain. The patient may be experiencing pain at a site distant to the surgical incision, not covered by the epidural analgesia, but still related to the surgery (e.g. shoulder tip pain after upper gastrointestinal or thoracic surgery). If this is the case additional analgesia may be required in the form of balanced analgesia, i.e. non-steroidal anti-inflammatory drugs (NSAIDs) +/– paracetemol on a regular, rather than as required (*pro re nata* (prn)), basis (Chapter 4). Despite the addition of these drugs, in some situations extra opioid analgesia (e.g. intravenous patient controlled analgesia (IV PCA)) may be necessary. In such cases it would be necessary to use a local anaesthetic only solution for the epidural infusion, thereby reducing the potential risk of opioid induced respiratory depression.

In situations where the unrelieved pain is related directly to the site of surgery, the following management strategies may be employed (Macintyre and Ready, 2001; South Wales Pain Nurses' Forum and Welsh Acute Pain Interest Group, 2002).

- Check the position of the epidural catheter and look for signs of leakage and/or displacement at site.
- Check for disconnection of the epidural line.
- Check that the device has not inadvertently been switched off.
- Administer a bolus dose of the epidural infusion and increase the rate of the infusion, within acceptable or prescribed parameters, and re-check the level of sensory block.
- Request a test dose or top-up of between 3 and 8 ml of local anaesthetic solution (e.g. 0.25% bupivacaine) to be administered by an anaesthetist or member of the acute pain team and then re-check the level of the sensory block. Improvement of a bilateral sensory block indicates the need for an increased infusion rate or concentration of local anaesthetic solution.
- If the sensory block is unilateral (i.e. effective on one side only) the catheter tip may have moved position into one of the intervertebral foramina. This may require withdrawal of the catheter by 1 to 2 cm (note timing of anti-coagulant administration – see Chapter 9), repositioning the patient to lie on the unaffected side and/or the administration of a larger bolus dose.
- If the top-up is ineffective the catheter is probably displaced, requiring reinsertion of the catheter (note timing of anticoagulant administration) or arrangements for alternative analgesia, e.g. IV PCA.

A recent prospective survey of 1062 patients receiving epidural analgesia in surgical wards reported that 20% of patients required reinsertion of the epidural catheter or alternative analgesic technique within 48 hours of initial catheter insertion (Burstal *et al.*, 1998a). The study's findings attributed approximately 50% of these failures to the accidental dislodgement of the catheter from the epidural space.

OPIOID AND/OR LOCAL ANAESTHETIC DRUG RELATED ADVERSE EFFECTS

Combinations of low concentrations of an opioid and a local anaesthetic are commonly used in an attempt to provide effective analgesia, while minimising the adverse effects of either drug. Drug related adverse effects may be separated into those activated by the opioid constituent (respiratory depression, sedation, nausea and vomiting, pruritis, urinary retention, hallucination) and those attributed to the local anaesthetic component (hypotension, dense motor or high sensory blockade, urinary retention, local anaesthetic toxicity, total spinal).

Opioid Induced Adverse Effects

All side effects of epidural opioids are mediated via opioid receptors; therefore treatment will often involve the administration of an opioid receptor antagonist, e.g. naloxone.

Respiratory Depression and Sedation

Respiratory depression is a major concern in epidural analgesia, it seems to be more of a problem with lipid insoluble drugs such as morphine, but has also occurred with the use of highly lipid soluble drugs, such as fentanyl. The early onset of this complication may be noted within minutes with lipid soluble opioids. In contrast, respiratory depression may occur within one hour after epidural morphine administration but could also occur up to 20 hours after epidural morphine is stopped, making late onset respiratory depression potentially more dangerous. Delayed respiratory depression is believed to be due to the rostral spread of the opioid in the CSF up to the medullary respiratory centre by diffusion and bulk flow (Rawal, 2003). Rather than a sudden event, respiratory depression has a slow and progressive onset, therefore continuous monitoring of sedation and respiratory rate is essential for the detection of late onset respiratory depression with lipid insoluble drugs.

Respiratory depression due to opioid analgesia occurs with similar frequency regardless of the route of delivery (i.e. intravenous or epidural). However, the systemic administration of opioid analgesia is associated more with sedation than with epidural delivery (Rathmell *et al.*, 2003). In a recent large study of epidural analgesia (Burstal *et al.*, 1998a), moderate to high levels of sedation occurred in 0.77% of patients, while respiratory depression occurred in 0.32% of patients, two from the fentanyl group and two from the morphine group. Three of the four episodes of respiratory depression were associated with sedation and all four patients required reversal with naloxone. There were no reported cases of delayed respiratory depression in this study.

Similar results were reported in the other large studies by de Leon-Casasola *et al.* (1994) and Scott *et al.* (1995) where the incidence of respiratory depression ranged from 0.07% to 1.2%, while the incidence of sedation occurred in 0.07% to 7.4% respectively. In the comparative study by Gedney and Liu (1998) the incidence of sedation and respiratory depression was reported on for five opioid–bupivacaine combinations. The incidence of sedation was low. No patients receiving diamorphine, methadone, fentanyl or pethidine became sedated and only one patient (0.6%) receiving morphine became sedated and respiratory depressed.

However, there are some studies reporting a higher incidence of respiratory depression with up to 10% of patients developing this complication (Weightman, 1991). High incidences of sedation and respiratory depression have been frequently associated with high doses of opioids, particularly by bolus (White *et al.*, 1992; Hayes *et al.*, 1993). This wide range may be related to the opioid used and the classification of respiratory depression, as studies vary in their definition of respiratory depression (i.e. a respiratory rate less than eight breaths per minute or a rate of less than ten breaths per minute). Respiratory depression should be characterised by a respiratory rate of less than eight breaths per minute and accompanied by an increased level of sedation.

Treatment includes stopping the epidural infusion, providing face mask oxygen (at 4 lpm), commencing IV administration of the opioid antagonist naloxone 100 μg at three to five minute intervals (to a maximum of 400 μg) until the respiratory rate is greater than 12 breaths per minute. The anaesthetist and/or a member of the acute pain service should be contacted to review the patient. Meticulous dose titration of naloxone administration is essential to avoid sudden reversal of analgesia. Also the short elimination half-life of naloxone may necessitate repeated IV injections or the administration of a continuous low dose infusion. It would be prudent to restart the epidural infusion at a reduced rate (25–50% reduction) and it may be appropriate to reduce or omit the opioid component in the epidural solution.

The clinical implications of this complication are for the routine provision of postoperative oxygen therapy, continuous monitoring of sedation and respiratory function, with the early intervention and treatment with naloxone when clinically indicated.

Hypotension

Sympathetic blockade, due to epidural local anaesthetic agents, can lead to hypotension as an effect of vasodilatation; there are implications for postoperative fluid management and patient monitoring for the early detection of this problem. Progressive hypovolaemia in the presence of an epidural block can result in severe and prolonged hypotension, cerebrovascular accident and myocardial infarction (Dawson, 1995).

In a recent meta-analysis (Block *et al.*, 2003) the incidence of hypotension with local anaesthetic based epidural infusions ranged from 8% to 14%, although the incidence of clinically relevant hypotension was believed to be higher in clinical practice. In a large study Burstal *et al.* (1998a) reported that hypotension occurred in 2.9% of patients, in comparison with other studies (Weightman, 1991; de Leon-Casasola *et al.*, 1994) where the incidence was reported to be 3% and 6.6% respectively. In contrast Gedney and Liu (1998) concluded that hypotension occurred in 17.5% of patients. In all of these patients the hypotension responded to fluids, vasoconstrictors were not required.

Therefore, the routine monitoring of blood pressure is essential in order to detect hypotension and its possible sequelae at an early stage, especially after bolus administration. The importance of this can be seen in one study (Kurek and Lagares-Garcia, 1997), where the incidence of hypotension increased from 3% for the continuous epidural infusion group to 8% for the bolus infusion group.

Effective management of this complication includes ensuring that a selection of IV fluids and vasopressor drugs is readily available in all areas employing epidural techniques. Firstly, the cause of the hypovolaemia should be established; if it is thought to be volume related an increase in the rate of IV fluid administration should be carried out. Contacting the acute pain service or anaesthetist is also essential as vasopressors (e.g. ephedrine) may be required in conjunction with fluid administration, especially if the hypotension is severe or if there has been little response to the increased IV fluids. Continued close monitoring is essential.

Dense and/or High Block

Dense lower limb blockade occurs more frequently with concentrated local anaesthetic solutions. It is also more consistent with lumbar epidural catheters used for lower limb and lower abdominal surgery, but can arise with thoracic epidurals. Dense blockade will impede mobility with a loss of proprioception or motor power.

In a recent meta-analysis (Block *et al.*, 2003) the incidence of lower extremity motor block, with postoperative epidural analgesia using local anaesthetic based solutions, ranged from 1% to 3%. However, in one large study (Burstal *et al.*, 1998a) leg weakness occurred in 8.4% of patients, whereas high sensory block was a reported problem for 1.3% of patients. There was an approximately 50% increase in the incidence of leg weakness related to the stronger 0.25% bupivacaine solution (14%), when compared with the 0.125% bupivacaine solution (7.6%). In another study (Kurek and Lagares-Garcia, 1997), the incidence of motor blockade and paraesthesia was reported as the most common adverse effect, occurring in 18% of patients with a continuous infusion of an opioid and bupivacaine 0.125% combination. This high incidence of leg weakness is of concern, and in contrast with the 3% reported in other studies achieving low levels of motor block by administration of appropriate doses of local anaesthetic is paramount (Bardra *et al.*, 1995).

The Bromage score is commonly used to monitor the effects of epidural analgesia on the motor power of the lower limbs (Bromage, 1978) and may be an early indicator for the first signs of catheter migration into CSF, or the presence of an epidural space haematoma/abscess. However, high sensory blockade may be a consequence of rostral spread of the local anaesthetic and may lead to patient complaints of weakness in upper limbs and varying degrees of motor block. The introduction of a scale, similar to the Bromage score, to monitor and control the upper level of high epidural blockade has been developed by Abd Elrazek and colleagues (1999). The ESSAM score enables easy and safe monitoring of thoracic epidurals, in order to avoid the risk of high cervical blockade, which may cause problems with respiration due to inadvertent blockade of diaphragmatic innervation. During the study period the scale proved to be sensitive in detecting the cranial–rostral spread early, giving staff the confidence to know and control the upper extension of motor blockade. An adaptation of this scoring system for thoracic epidurals in other surgical specialities has been implemented into clinical practice (Table 10.4).

Nausea and Vomiting

Nausea and vomiting are commonly encountered side effects of epidural opioids and may be due to a systemic effect, especially with lipid soluble opioids. Alternatively it may be due to rostral spread of the opioid in the CSF and interaction with opioid receptors in the area postrema. In part the actions of opioids on sensitisation of the vestibular system to motion and decreased gastric emptying also have a causative effect (Rawal, 2003).

A recent meta-analysis reports the cumulative incidence of nausea and vomiting, in patients receiving continuous infusions of epidural opioids, to be as high as 45–80% (Block *et al.*, 2003). In one large study (Burstal *et al.*, 1998a) of epidural fentanyl–bupivacaine analgesia, nausea and vomiting were reported to be a problem for 2.8% of patients compared with 3.1% of patients reported by Scott *et al.* (1995). However, in other large studies (Ready *et al.*, 1991; de Leon-Casasola *et al.*, 1994) the incidence of nausea and vomiting increased to 29% and 22% respectively. But, even with the highly lipid soluble opioids some studies report incidences of nausea and vomiting to be as high as 25–35% (Kurek and Lagares-Garcia, 1997).

In the comparative study by Gedney and Liu (1998), the incidence of nausea and vomiting was reported for five opioid–bupivacaine combinations. This study found nausea was a common side effect occurring in 54% of all patients. Morphine had the highest incidence and severity of nausea (78%) and vomiting (47%), and patients were twice as likely to experience nausea with morphine than with fentanyl and methadone. The incidence of nausea and vomiting with morphine has been shown to be dose dependent (Crawford *et al.*, 1981).

Antiemetics are commonly prescribed for the treatment and prophylaxis of nausea and vomiting, however unwanted sedation from some antiemetics may exacerbate respiratory depression (Rawal, 2003). Treatment of nausea and vomiting depends on severity; the implementation of a guide and algorithm for the administration of regular antiemetics may prove beneficial, thereby improving the overall management of this distressing complication (see Figure 10.1).

In studies, subhypnotic doses of propofol have been reported to reduce nausea and vomiting (Gedney and Liu, 1998), while IV dexamethasone has also been shown to be beneficial in preventing postoperative nausea and vomiting (PONV) after epidural morphine (Ho *et al.*, 2001).

Pruritis

The mechanism of pruritis (itching) is not fully understood, it does not appear to be dependent on histamine release and may be a symptom of local excitation of opioid receptors within the spinal cord (Rawal, 2003). However, pruritis is reported to be one of the most common adverse effects from epidural administration of opioids with an overall incidence of approximately 60%, compared with the incidence of 15% for those patients receiving systemic opioids (Block *et al.*, 2003).

The reported incidence of pruritis varies considerably from study to study and the probable reason for this is that the majority of patients do not complain about this complication because of its mild nature. With morphine the incidence of pruritis varies from 0% to 100%, for diamorphine and fentanyl 5% to 75%, for methadone 0% to 9% and for pethidine 13% to 59% (Gedney and Liu, 1998). In one large study (Burstal *et al.*, 1998a) pruritis was reported to be a problem for 2.4% of patients; although there was a likelihood of under-reporting as only those patients requiring treatment were recorded. The highest incidence was seen in the lumbar morphine epidural group, with 8.8% of patients reporting pruritis to be a problem. Other large studies of patients receiving epidural morphine analgesia have reported incidences of 22% and 11% respectively (Ready *et al.*, 1991; de Leon-Casasola *et al.*, 1994). This is in comparison with the 10.3% incidence for pruritus reported by Scott *et al.* (1995) using fentanyl–bupivacaine infusions.

In one recent study (Ready *et al.*, 1991) pruritis occurred in 29% of patients. Morphine and diamorphine had the same incidence of pruritis (44%), which was significantly higher than that of methadone (12.5%) and pethidine (15.6%). However, the study found that of the 15.6% of patients receiving

- PONV can have many causes. Try to minimise pain, ensure rest and adequate hydration
- Encourage patients to inform staff at an early stage if they feel nauseous
- PONV can cause dehydration, electrolyte imbalance, disrupt surgical wounds and slow recovery
- Try to identify those at most risk of PONV and treat prophylactically for the first 24–48 hours postoperatively; e.g. one drug regular and another PRN from a different drug group
- Assess 4-hourly or more frequently if required

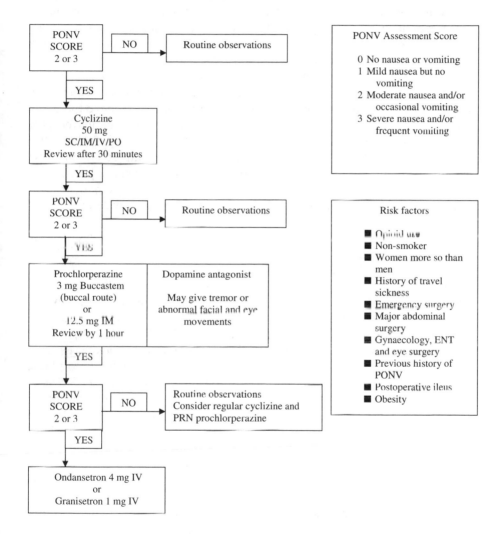

Figure 10.1. Algorithm for managing nausea and vomiting – a guide to the management of postoperative nausea and vomiting (PONV). (From an original idea of Dr D. Counsell at South Wales Pain Nurses' Forum.)

pethidine and experiencing pruritis, the itching was so severe the infusion had to be stopped in 80% of these patients.

In patients with epidural analgesia pruritis is often generalised but more likely to be localised to the face, neck and upper thorax. Epidural fentanyl is more likely to cause segmental pruritis, whereas epidural morphine is associated with generalised itching (Rawal, 2003). Facial itching results from opioid ascent in CSF to the third and fourth ventricle, while itch in immunocompromised patients with a history of cold sores may result in herpes simplex reactivation; 75% of patients receiving epidural morphine developed pruritis with reactivation of herpes simplex (Dawson, 1995).

Treatment of pruritis depends on severity. In mild cases no treatment, or simply reducing the opioid concentration in the infusion, may be required. In severe cases 50–100 μg of intravenous naloxone can help to relieve the effect (Gedney and Liu, 1998) suggesting the existence of an opioid receptor mediated central mechanism. Subhypnotic doses (10 mg) of propofol have also been shown to relieve morphine induced pruritis (Rawal, 2003). In some instances antiemetic and antihistaminic drugs are used to manage pruritis, but are generally seen as ineffective and have the potential to add to patient sedation (Dawson, 1995). Intractable pruritis may necessitate removal of the opioid from the epidural infusion.

Urinary Retention/Incontinence

Epidural opioid induced urinary retention is likely to be related to interaction with opioid receptors located in the sacral spinal cord, promoting inhibition of sacral parasympathetic nervous system outflow, which causes detrusor muscle relaxation and an increase in bladder capacity (Rawal, 2003).

The incidence of urinary retention following epidural opioids varies considerably, but is known to be greater in patients receiving epidural morphine, ranging from 10% to 100%. In one recent study of orthopaedic patients receiving lumbar epidural infusions conducted by Gedney and Liu (1998) morphine was associated with a significantly greater incidence of urinary retention than pethidine and methadone. Patients receiving morphine were more likely to require catheterisation (76%) than those receiving methadone (39%) and pethidine (35%). In total 71% of all patients in this study were catheterised. However, in a previous study (Reay et al., 1989) 40% of orthopaedic patients required catheterisation after a non-opioid spinal anaesthetic and no epidural. The incidence of urinary retention following epidural diamorphine and fentanyl is unknown.

Naloxone has been shown to reduce this side effect of epidural opioids (Gedney and Liu, 1998), although the usual doses used for reversal of respiratory depression may be inadequate to reverse urinary retention. Treatment of urinary retention is catheterisation and some would advocate a single 'in and out' catheter to reduce the possibility of infection. Catheterisation with possible bacteraemia may lead to prosthesis infection in patients undergoing hip and knee arthroplasty. Nevertheless, if a patient is unable to void urine six hours after surgery catheterisation is indicated to prevent potential bladder damage due to over-distension (Rawal, 2003).

Hallucination

Hallucinations can occasionally occur with the administration of opioids. In one large study (Burstal *et al.*, 1998a) of epidural analgesia, 0.31% of patients reported hallucination as an adverse effect. The severity of this complication is often mild, but if the patient is distressed, the healthcare professional should reassure them and explain why it is happening and advice should be sought from the acute pain service. If the epidural analgesia is providing effective pain relief, but the patient is experiencing unacceptable adverse effects, it may be possible to improve the situation. Consideration should be given to the administration of regular balanced analgesia, i.e. paracetemol +/– NSAIDs, with a decrease in the rate of the epidural infusion and altering the prescription accordingly. However, it may be necessary to change the opioid or remove it from the epidural infusion entirely.

Local Anaesthetic Toxicity

High blood concentration of local anaesthetic agents can lead to systemic toxicity and may occur if excessive doses are given or if a therapeutic dose is inadvertently injected into an epidural blood vessel (Macintyre and Ready, 2001). Toxicity caused by local anaesthetics may manifest differently according to the drug used. It results from the effects of the local anaesthetic on the central nervous system and the cardiovascular system (CVS). Early signs and symptoms of central nervous system toxicity will present with the patient reporting light-headedness, numbness of mouth and tongue and ringing in the ears. This will progress to visual and auditory disturbances, muscle twitches, unconsciousness, convulsions, coma, respiratory arrest, bradycardia and cardiac arrest if the blood concentration continues to rise (Kingsley, 2001; Macintyre and Ready, 2001).

It is vital to treat the early signs and symptoms promptly and effectively to prevent the progression of complications. Treatment depends on the stage and severity of toxicity and requires relevant supportive management at each stage, e.g. oxygenation, anticonvulsants, intubation and ventilation, cardiac resuscitation.

EQUIPMENT RELATED ADVERSE EFFECTS

LEAKAGE FROM THE EPIDURAL CATHETER INSERTION SITE

Leakage of the epidural analgesic solution from the insertion site does not always necessitate the need to abandon the epidural. If pain is well controlled the epidural should be continued and the leakage documented. Continued monitoring of the patient is essential to detect a worsening situation. Should the patient experience moderate to severe levels of pain the following is advised.

- Test the height of the sensory block.
- Check the epidural catheter distance markings – ascertain if the catheter has moved out of position since insertion.
- Contact the acute pain service or anaesthetist to review the problem and consider giving an epidural bolus dose (see Figure 10.2).
- Consider removing the epidural catheter; either re-site the epidural or provide an alternative method of analgesia, e.g. IV PCA.

Disconnection of the Epidural Catheter from the Antibacterial Filter

Fixation of the epidural antibacterial filter to the patient's anterior chest wall or shoulder may reduce the potential occurrence of this problem (see Figure 10.3). Disconnection of the antibacterial filter puts the patient at high risk of infection, therefore best practice dictates the immediate removal of the epidural catheter to prevent further complications. The practice of trimming the end of the epidural catheter and attaching a new filter is no longer advisable. The acute pain service or anaesthetist will need to be informed, as alternative analgesia or re-siting of the epidural may be indicated.

Epidural Catheter Dislodgement

Accidental dislodgement of epidural catheters is a consistently reported problem, which has a recognised impact on the provision of reliable analgesia in patients with epidurals. Careful attention needs to be given to the epidural catheter during patient movement, positioning and mobilisation in order to avoid this problem.

In one large study Burstal *et al.* (1998a) reported the necessity for premature removal of epidural catheters due to accidental dislodgement in 13% of their patient population. Other studies have shown that catheter dislodgement accounts for epidural analgesia failure in 1.6–12.6% of patients (de Leon-Casasola *et al.*, 1994). In the obstetric population, Phillips and MacDonald (1987) reported an incidence of up to 50% of catheters moving

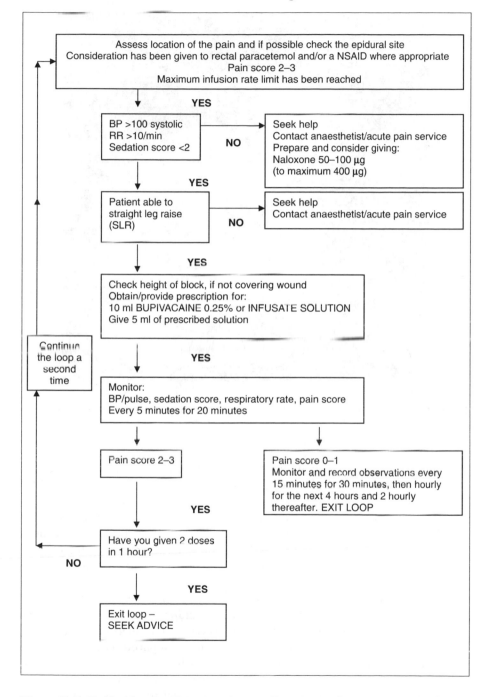

Figure 10.2. Epidural top-up flow chart for unrelieved pain. (South Wales Pain Nurses' Forum – 2002 unpublished)

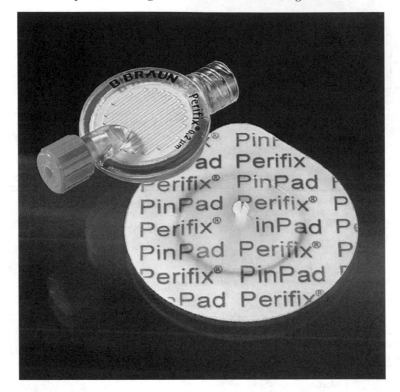

Figure 10.3. Antibacterial filter fixative device. (Reproduced by permission of B-Braun Medical Ltd.)

from their original position, while this problem has also been documented in thoracic epidurals used for postoperative patients by Mourisse *et al.* (1989).

In a recent large study (Clark *et al.*, 2001) of postoperative patients receiving epidural analgesia, analgesic failure was reported in 16% of patients due to outward catheter migration. The method of fixation was the commonly used technique of coiling the catheter under a transparent dressing (Duffy, 1981) and in another study accounted for 36% of outward catheter migration in obstetric patients (Bishton *et al.*, 1992).

Conversely, Burstal *et al.* (1998b) reported a significant reduction in the migration of the epidural catheter with the subcutaneous tunnelling technique. This randomised controlled trial (RCT) showed a reduction for outward migration of just 10% in their tunnelled group compared with 29% in the standard group and also no movement at all of the catheter in 86% of their tunnelled group compared with 67% of their standard group. However, the tunnelling method is invasive and has the potential for the development of additional risks, such as bleeding, catheter damage and inflammation at the subcutaneous tunnel site. Tripathi and Pandey (2000) also used a tunnelled technique and reported a 27% incidence of inflammation around the tunnel site.

Clark *et al.* (2001) investigated the efficacy of using the 'Lockit' epidural catheter clamp in preventing epidural catheter migration. They reported no movement at the insertion site in 88% of the study group compared with 28% in the standard group (coiled catheter under a transparent dressing). Outward migration greater than 2 cm occurred in 26% of the standard group compared with 6% of the study group and inward migration of 1 cm occurred in 17% of the standard group compared with none in the study group. They concluded that these results compared favourably with the studies on tunnelling and suggest this approach avoids the more complicated and invasive method of catheter fixation. Several other non-invasive methods of epidural catheter fixation have been tested in clinical practice in an attempt to prevent catheter dislodgement (Lawler and Anderson, 2002).

Sheared off Epidural Catheter Tip

The occurrence of a sheared off epidural catheter tip is extremely rare. Best practice dictates that anaesthetists should never withdraw the catheter back through the epidural needle if there is a problem, i.e. a dural tap at the time of insertion, as there is a likelihood of shearing off the tip. However, if the epidural catheter tip is sheared off this must be noted in the patient's medical and nursing records, reported to the senior duty anaesthetist and the patient's clinical team, and the patient must be fully informed of the event and possible consequences. The sheared off catheter will not cause any problems within the epidural space, the patient will not experience any lasting effects and surgical intervention to remove the catheter is unnecessary.

Epidural Infusion Device

Erroneous problems with epidural infusion devices include the mis-programming of pumps, malfunctioning of pumps, probable patient tampering and interference with the device along with incorrect drug/fluid administration through the device or epidural line. Clear labelling of epidural infusion devices, catheters and administration lines is essential to reduce the occurrence of human error (Chapter 5).

Burstal *et al.* (1998a) reported five cases of error in the administration of the epidural infusion. On two occasions a bolus of 200 ml of the infusion solution was given due to neglecting to set a limit on the infusion pump – it had been intended to give only a 5–10 ml bolus from the bag. One patient developed a very high sensory block and the other developed mild hypotension, both of which responded to treatment. The other cases were similar but the volumes infused were much smaller and did not result in any systemic effects.

Patient fatalities have been attributed to the incorrect programming of epidural infusion pumps by healthcare staff not adequately trained in the setting up and programming of the device. Formal competency based training programmes are essential for maintaining patient safety and minimising the risks associated with epidural infusion devices. The importance of equipment choice for the delivery of epidural infusions is discussed in Chapter 5, while education and competency are considered in Chapter 11.

In conclusion, there is a significant number of adverse effects associated with postoperative epidural analgesia, which necessitate a risk–benefit analysis in the decision to use the technique for a given patient population (Chapter 2). Studies (Gedney and Liu, 1998) have shown that up to 25% of patients with epidural analgesia have good pain relief without any adverse effects.

The low incidence of major complications (1 in 2000 to 1 in 10000) (Giebler *et al.*, 1997) can be achieved by an integrated team approach to the management of epidural analgesia. Emphasis on prompt recognition and treatment of adverse effects is essential.

REFERENCES

Abaza, K. and Bogod, D. (2004) Cerebrospinal fluid–cutaneous fistula and pseudomonas meningitis complicating thoracic epidural analgesia. *British Journal of Anaesthesia*, **92**, 429–31.

Abd Elrazek, E., Scott, N. and Vohra, A. (1999) An epidural scoring scale for arm movements [ESSAM] in patients receiving high thoracic epidural analgesia for coronary artery bypass grafting. *Anaesthesia*, **54**, 1097–109.

Abouleish, E. and Goldstein, M. (1986) Migration of an extra-dural catheter into the subdural space. *British Journal of Anaesthesia*, **58**, 1194–7.

Aldrete, J., Daniel, W., O'Higgins, J. *et al.* (1971) Analysis of anaesthetic-related morbidity in human recipients of renal homo-grafts. *Anesthesia & Analgesia*, **50**, 321–9.

Bardra, L., Funch-Jensen, P., Crawford, M. and Kehlet, H. (1995) Recovery after laparascopic colonic surgery with epidural analgesia, and early oral nutrition and mobilisation. *Lancet*, **345**, 763–4.

Basta, M. and Sloan, P. (1999) Epidural haematoma following epidural catheter placement in a patient with chronic renal failure. *Canadian Journal of Anesthesia*, **46**, 271–4.

Bishton, I., Martin, P., Vernon, J. and Liu, W. (1992) Factors influencing epidural catheter migration. *Anaesthesia*, **47**, 610–12.

Block, M., Liu, S., Rowlingson, A. *et al.* (2003) Efficacy of postoperative epidural analgesia. Meta-analysis. *Journal of the American Medical Association*, **290**, 2455–63.

Bougher, R., Corbett, A. and Ramage, D. (1996) The effect of tunnelling on epidural catheter migration. *Anaesthesia*, **51**, 191–4.

Bromage, P. (1978) *Epidural Analgesia*. London: WB Saunders.

Burstal, R., Wegener, F., Hayes, C. and Langtry, G. (1998a) Epidural analgesia: prospective audit of 1062 patients. *Anaesthesia and Intensive Care*, **26**, 165–72.

Burstal, R., Wegener, F. Hayes, C. and Langtry, G. (1998b) Subcutaneous tunnelling of epidural catheters for postoperative analgesia – a randomised controlled trial. *Anaesthesia*, **51**, 191–4.

Clark, M., O'Hare, K., Gorringe, J. and Oh, T. (2001) The effect of the Lockit epidural catheter clamp on epidural migration: a controlled trial. *Anaesthesia*, **56**, 865–70.

Crawford, R., Batra, M. and Fox, F. (1981) Epidural morphine dose response for postoperative analgesia. *Anaesthesiology*, **55**, A150.

Dawson, P. (1995) Postoperative epidural analgesia. *Current Anaesthesia and Critical Care*, **6**, 69–75.

de Leon-Casasola, O., Parker, B., Lema, M. *et al.* (1994) Postoperative epidural bupivacaine–morphine therapy: experience with 4227 surgical cancer patients. *Anaesthesiology*, **81**, 368–75.

Duffy, B. (1981) Epidural catheter fixation. *Anaesthesia and Intensive Care*, **9**, 292.

Gedney, J. and Liu, E. (1998) Side effects of epidural infusions of opioid bupivacaine mixtures. *Anaesthesia*, **53**, 1148–55.

Giebler, M. (1997) Incidence of neurological complications related to thoracic epidural catheterisation. *Anaesthesiology*, **86**, 55–63.

Giebler, R., Scherer, R. and Peters, J. (1997) Incidence of neurological complications related to thoracic epidural catheterisation. *Anaesthesiology*, **86**, 55–63.

Hayes, S., Davidson, I., Allsop, J. and Dutton, D. (1993) Comparison of epidural methadone with epidural diamorphine for analgesia following caesarean section. *Acta Anaesthesiology Scandinavia*, **38**, 328–35.

Ho, S., Wang, J. and Tzeng, J. (2001) Dexamethasone for preventing nausea and vomiting associated with epidural morphine: a dose ranging study. *Anesthesia & Analgesia*, **92**, 745–8.

Horlocker, T., Wedel, D. and Schroder, D. (1995) Preoperative anti-platelet therapy does not increase the risk of spinal haematoma associated with regional anaesthesia. *Anesthesia & Analgesia*, **80**, 303–9.

Horlocker, T., Wedel, D., Benzon, H. *et al.* (2003) Regional anaesthesia in the anticoagulated patient: defining the risks (the second ASRA consensus conference on neuraxial anaesthesia and anticoagulation). *Regional Anaesthesia and Pain Medicine*, **28**, 172–97.

Justins, D. (2004) Good practice in continuous epidural analgesia for acute pain management. *Royal College of Anaesthetists Bulletin*, **26**, 1309–12.

Kindler, C., Seeberger, M. and Staender, S. (1998) Epidural abscess complicating epidural anaesthesia and analgesia. *Acta Anaesthesiology Scandinavia*, **42**, 614–20.

Kingsley, C. (2001) Epidural analgesia, your role. *Registered Nurse*, **64** (3), 53–8.

Kurek, S. and Lagares-Garcia, J. (1997) Complications of epidural infusions for analgesia in postoperative and trauma patients. *American Surgeon*, **63**, 543–6.

Lawler, K. and Anderson, T. (2002) Regional trial of five epidural fixation products and a commonly used 'control'. *Pain Network Newsletter*, No. 32. http://www.painnetwork.co.uk.html (accessed 20.08.04).

Macintyre, P. and Ready, L. (2001) *Acute Pain Management: A Practical Guide*, 2nd edn. London: W B Saunders.

Mourisse, M., Gielen, M. and Hasenbos, M. (1989) Migration of thoracic epidural catheters: three methods for evaluation of catheter position in the thoracic epidural space. *Anaesthesia*, **44**, 574–7.

O'Higgins, F. and Tuckey, J. (2000) Thoracic epidural anaesthesia and analgesia: United Kingdom practice. *Acta Anaesthesiology Scandinavia*, **44**, 1087–92.

Phillips, D. and MacDonald, R. (1987) Epidural catheter migration during labour. *Anaesthesia*, **54**, 98–9.

Phillips, D., MacDonald, R. and Lyons, G. (1986) Possible sub-arachnoid migration of an epidural catheter. *Anaesthesia*, **41**, 653–4.

Rathmell, J., Neal, J. and Liu, S. (2003) Outcome measures in acute pain management. In: Rowbotham, D. and MacIntyre, P. (eds). *Clinical Pain Management. Acute Pain*. London: Arnold.

Ravindran, R., Albrecht, W. and McKay, M. (1979) Apparent intra-vascular migration of epidural catheter. *Anesthesia & Analgesia*, **58**, 252–3.

Rawal, N. (2003) Intra-spinal opioids. In: Rowbotham, D. and MacIntyre, P. (eds). *Clinical Pain Management. Acute Pain*. London: Arnold.

Ready, L., Loper, K., Nessly, M. and Wild, L. (1991) Postoperative epidural morphine is safe on surgical wards. *Anaesthesiology*, **75**, 452–6.

Reay, B., Semple, A., Macrae, W. *et al.* (1989) Low dose intrathecal diamorphine analgesia following major orthopaedic surgery. *British Journal of Anaesthesia*, **62** (3), 248–52.

Scott, D., Beiby, S. and McClymont, C. (1995) Postoperative epidural analgesia using epidural infusions of fentanyl with bupivacaine. *Anaesthesiology*, **83**, 727–37.

Scottish Intercollegiate Guidelines Network (2004) Prophylaxis of venous thromboembolism. Section 7: Spinal and epidural block. http://www.sign.ac.uk/guidelines/fulltext/62/section7.html (accessed 20.08.04).

South Wales Pain Nurses' Forum (SWPNF) and Welsh Acute Pain Interest Group (WAPIG) (2002) Epidural Analgesia in Adult Acute Pain Management: Best Practice Guidelines for the Region of South Wales. Unpublished.

South Wales Pain Nurses' Forum (SWPNF) and Welsh Acute Pain Interest Group (WAPIG) (2003) Intravenous patient controlled analgesia in adult acute pain management: Best practice guidelines for the region of South Wales. Unpublished.

Steffan, P., Seeling, W., Essig, A. *et al.* (2004) Bacterial contamination of epidural catheters: microbiological examination of 502 epidural catheters used for postoperative analgesia. *Journal of Clinical Anaesthesia*, **16**, 92–7.

Swansea Acute Pain Management Service (2004) Multidisciplinary guidelines for epidural analgesia in postoperative pain management (adults) 16 years and over. Unpublished.

Tripathi, M. and Pandey, M. (2000) Epidural catheter fixation: subcutaneous tunnelling with a loop to prevent displacement. *Anaesthesia*, **55**, 1141–2.

Wang, P. (1999) Incidence of spinal epidural abscess after epidural analgesia. *Anaesthesiology*, **91**, 1928–36.

Weightman, W. (1991) Respiratory arrest during epidural infusion of bupivacaine and fentanyl. *Anesthesia & Analgesia*, **19**, 282–4.

White, M., Berghausen, E. and Dumont, S. (1992) Side effects during continuous epidural infusion of morphine and fentanyl. *Canadian Journal of Anaesthesia*, **39**, 576–82.

Williams, B. and Wheatley, R. (2000) Epidural analgesia for postoperative pain relief. *Royal College of Anaesthetists Bulletin*, **2**, 68–71.

Wulf, H. (1996) Epidural anaesthesia and spinal haematoma. *Canadian Journal of Anesthesia*, **12**, 1260–71.

11

Education and Training

CAROLYN MIDDLETON

Clinical Nurse Specialist in Pain Management, Nevill Hall Hospital,
Abergavenny, South Wales

Education and training have become central to the delivery of the modernisation agenda for the NHS (DoH, 1999a). The overall training strategy for a trust must ensure that healthcare professionals are equipped with the appropriate knowledge base and competencies required to meet the needs of the service.

This chapter aims to provide an overview of the competency based training required for healthcare professionals in relation to epidural analgesia along with a framework describing how the training might fit into the Agenda for Change, Knowledge and Skills framework. A brief overview of patient education in relation to epidurals will also be provided.

EDUCATION AND TRAINING

The safe management and troubleshooting of epidural infusions requires skill and knowledge, therefore every hospital that uses epidural infusions should have an ongoing programme to meet the educational needs of nursing and other members of the multidisciplinary healthcare team.

First of all it is necessary to identify the learning needs of the target population so that an appropriate programme of learning can be developed. The education and training must take account of statutory and/or mandatory

Epidural Analgesia in Acute Pain Management. Edited by Carolyn Middleton.
© 2006 by John Wiley & Sons, Ltd.   ISBN 0-470-01964-6

requirements (for example health and safety regulations dictate that it is a statutory requirement for staff to be appropriately trained to use infusion devices). The programme must also take account of clinical governance issues such as risk management and clinical incident reporting and must utilise evidence based practice.

Provisional plans for education should be discussed with the local training and development department for the trust; once agreement has been reached the plans can be finalised and implemented. Training should utilise workplace learning, internally run education and training programmes, local university courses and other external education providers. Some training can take the form of 'E-learning', online theoretical learning packages which can incorporate an assessment of attained knowledge. This sort of learning can be developed to meet local need, it is easily accessible to all staff who have access to a computer and offers a flexible schedule for undertaking learning as it is always available for use night and day.

Education relating to epidural practice should encompass the broad principles that have been presented in this book.

- Responsibilities of the multidisciplinary team in relation to epidural infusions.
- Patient selection, risk–benefit analysis and issues relating to informed consent.
- Anatomy of the epidural space and the principles of catheter insertion.
- The physiology of acute pain, pharmacodynamics and pharmacokinetics of local anaesthetics and opioids and general principles of prescribing in relation to epidural infusions.
- Epidural delivery systems, i.e. equipment, modes of delivery and documentation.
- Patient observations and epidural infusion device monitoring and documentation.
- Discontinuation of epidural infusions and removal of the epidural catheter.
- Troubleshooting, recognising and treating adverse effects.
- Clinical governance and clinical audit.

Service priorities must be considered when organising an education programme and dependent on the target population for education it may also be necessary to include specific content relating to epidural infusion use in obstetrics and/or paediatric practice. Issues of feasibility of release of staff from the clinical area should be taken into account when planning the length and number of sessions that individual staff will be required to attend.

Unqualified staff also play a vital role (both directly and indirectly) in the care delivered to patients receiving epidural analgesia. Therefore, training at an appropriate level should be put into place to meet their specific needs.

COMPETENCY BASED DEVICE TRAINING

The push for greater accountability in health care has led to a greater emphasis on establishing baseline standards of acceptable performance recognised by individual regulatory bodies (Redman *et al.*, 1999). Maintaining professional standards by assessing competence helps individual nurses and trusts to provide safeguards for the general population and to protect themselves from the increasing culture of litigation and compensation (McMullan *et al.*, 2003; Fordham, 2005).

All staff, doctors, registered nurses and midwives and medical technicians who use epidural devices must receive appropriate training and be in possession of a valid assessment of competence certificate. Following assessment it is the responsibility of the user to ensure their continued competence in the use of the device. Individuals also have a responsibility to ensure they keep an up to date record of training undertaken and assessment of competence completed. It may be appropriate to record this information in a professional profile. Centrally within a trust's training and development department there should be records kept of all staff that have successfully completed competency based epidural device training.

There are many definitions of competence and competencies in the literature. The Nursing and Midwifery Council (NMC) defines competence in its Code of Professional Conduct as 'Possessing the skills and abilities required for lawful, safe and effective professional practice without direct supervision' (NMC, 2002). The competency based assessment approach is best suited to epidural training because by using competencies, performance of an individual can be effectively measured against a clearly defined set of outcomes. As the ultimate clinical practice goal is to evaluate performance for the effective application of knowledge and skills in the practice setting, these outcome measures provide clear evidence of ability or failure to perform manipulation of the epidural device (Redman *et al.*, 1999).

The assessment format should be consistent and standardised to ensure reliability and to provide assurance of comparable standards (see Table 11.1) (Fordham, 2005).

KNOWLEDGE AND SKILLS FRAMEWORK (KSF) AND AGENDA FOR CHANGE

Irrespective of how learning is delivered, increasingly healthcare professionals want to know how any material or developmental activity will relate to the KSF, thereby seeing clearly how it helps them to progress from one level to the next within the agenda for change pay structure.

Table 11.1. Extract from a competency based assessment

Performance criteria	Date	Attained	Referred	Signature of assessor
1. Inspection of pump				
(a) State clinical application of the pump				
(b) Explain the safety checks and precautions to be taken prior to using the pump				
(c) Identify the appropriate equipment needed for use with the pump				
2. Loading the cassette				
Demonstrate how to:				
(a) Attach cassette to external reservoir of epidural solution				
(b) Prime line through cassette				
(c) Insert cassette into pump				
(d) Load pump and reservoir into lock box				
3. Programming the 9500 pump				
(a) State the function of all the soft keys				
(b) Demonstrate how to switch on the pump				
(c) Explain the purpose of the pump self test				

The KSF applies to all healthcare staff (except doctors, dentists and some senior board members), it is a broad generic framework that defines and describes the knowledge and skills that staff need to apply in their work in order to deliver quality care to patients. It also provides a consistent comprehensive and explicit framework on which to base staff development.

For each role it will be necessary to have a fully developed KSF post outline that represents the knowledge and skills required to meet the needs of that post. Each post outline will include the six core KSF dimensions (communication; personal and people development; health, safety and security; service improvement; quality; equality and diversity) along with up to seven of the other 24 specific dimensions which are categorised under four headings: health and well-being; estates and facilities; information and knowledge; general (NHS Wales, 2004).

Table 11.2. KSF HWB7 dimension levels

1. Assist in providing interventions and/or treatments
2. Contribute to planning, delivering and monitoring interventions and/or treatments
3. Plan, deliver and evaluate interventions and/or treatments
4. Plan, deliver and evaluate interventions and/or treatments when there are complex issues and serious illness

For each dimension it will be necessary to determine the level and indicators that best describe the knowledge and skills needed to match the post. Individuals' work will be mapped against the KSF outline for their particular post, and each practitioner will be required to systematically gather valid, reliable and relevant evidence to support the fact that they have to meet the needs of each dimension (NHS Wales, 2004).

So for qualified nurses working within surgical wards or departments where epidural infusions are frequently utilised, one of the specific dimensions set out for their post may well be dimension HWB7 (health and well-being 7). Therefore, competency based training and assessment educational programmes need to be mapped to the specific needs of the KSF HWB7 dimension (Table 11.2).

For most registered nurses either a level 2 or 3 would be most appropriate. There may be some degree of planning and information given regarding epidural infusions that would take place with the patient preoperatively. Participation in the delivery and monitoring of the epidural infusion postoperatively would be a major part of the registered nurses' role and most nurses would also be taking an active role in evaluation of the efficacy of the epidural infusion and its associated adverse effects.

In the NHS knowledge and skills framework document (NHS Wales, 2004) it is suggested that progression through the levels in dimension HWB7 is characterised by complex procedures with high levels of associated risk, which require increasing levels of clinical and technical skills and knowledge. This dimension is guided by UK legislation such as health and safety laws (Chapter 5), the practice and regulation of particular professional bodies (Chapter 2) and also by local policy and guidelines.

Level 2 of the KSF HWB7 dimension is to contribute to planning, delivery and monitoring of interventions and/or treatments. Some of the relevant indicators set out in the KSF document for this level (NHS Wales, 2004) can be found in the left hand column of Table 11.3, with possible examples of application in the column on the right.

At level 3 of the KSF HWB7 dimension the above information still applies, but there are additional requirements set out in Table 11.4.

Table 11.3. KSF HWB7. An example of level 2 indicators and possible application relating to epidural infusion

Indicators	Possible application
1. Identify any specific precautions or contraindications to the proposed intervention and take the relevant action	Be aware of the indications and contraindications for epidural infusion. Inform the senior nurse or pain team of any concerns or relevant information
2. Prepare for, undertake and record interventions or treatments correctly and in line with legislation, policies and procedures and/or established protocols	Be aware of the responsibilities of the registered nurse in relation to all aspects of epidural infusions including documentation. Be familiar with national legislation and local policies and guidelines guiding the use of epidural infusions (Chapter 1).
3. Support and monitor people throughout promptly alerting the relevant person when there are unexpected changes in an individual's health and well-being or risks	Undertake a course of study which provides the individual with the appropriate knowledge base of the anatomy of the epidural space, epidural catheter insertion techniques (Chapter 3), knowledge of the pharmacokinetics and pharmacodynamics of the drugs used in epidural infusions and the modes of deliver (Chapters 4 and 5). Be aware of the appropriate monitoring required for a patient receiving an epidural infusion (Chapter 8) and be able to recognise deviations from the norm (Chapter 10). Undertake a competency based assessment for manipulation of the epidural device
4. Provide information to the team on how an individual's needs are changing and feedback on the appropriateness of the individual's treatment plan when there are issues	Demonstrate an appropriate level of both written and verbal communication and be able to recognise efficacy and potential adverse events associated with epidural infusions
5. Respond to, record and report any adverse events or incidents relating to the intervention or treatment with an appropriate degree or urgency	Undertake a course of study, which enables the practitioner to recognise complications and take appropriate action to minimise the risks for the patient (Chapter 10).

Table 11.4. KSF HWB7. An example of level 3 indicators and possible application relating to epidural infusion

Indicators	Possible application
1. Take account of the individual's physiological and/or psychological functioning	Undertake an appropriate course of study to enable the practitioner to perform a bio/psycho/social assessment of a patient prior to receiving an epidural infusion
The nature of the different aspects of the intervention and any specific precautions or contraindications to the proposed intervention	Undertake an appropriate course of study to be able to participate in a risk–benefit analysis of the patient considered for epidural infusion (Chapter 2). Be aware of risk management issues
The involvement of other people or agencies involved	Be aware of the agencies involved in the epidural infusion management and each practitioner's individual role (Chapter 1). Be aware of legislation, policies and procedures
2. Undertake the intervention in a manner that is consistent with evidence based practice and/or clinical guidelines	Be aware of the body of evidence that supports the use of epidural infusions (Chapters 4 and 5) as well as the national legislation and local policies and guidelines guiding the use of epidural infusions (Chapter 1)
Undertake the intervention through multidisciplinary team working	Participate in multidisciplinary team working regarding the epidural infusion, i.e. collaborative working with the pain team, anaesthetists, pharmacy, surgeons, EBME and heads of nursing (Chapter 1)
Undertake the intervention in a manner consistent with his or her own knowledge, skills and experience	Undertake a course of study which includes specific learning about epidural infusions. Maintain that level of knowledge and attend regular updates. Undertake a competency based assessment for manipulation of the epidural device
Undertake the intervention in a manner consistent with legislation, policies and procedures	Be familiar with all guidance documents relating to the safe use of epidural infusions
3. Review the effectiveness of the intervention and makes any necessary modifications	Be able to monitor efficacy of the epidural infusion and in the case of continuous-only infusions adjust the rate of infusion in line with efficacy and adverse reactions (Chapter 10)
Provide feedback to the person responsible for the overall treatment plan on its effectiveness	Communicate and liaise effectively with all members of the multidisciplinary team involved in the safe delivery of epidural infusions (Chapter 1)
4. Make accurate records of the interventions and outcomes	Ensure that documentation meets the legal requirements at all times (Chapters 1 and 5)

The outcomes following the undertaking of such formal study should be that individuals have gained new knowledge and skills, developed themselves and are better equipped to apply their knowledge and skills to their clinical practice.

PATIENT EDUCATION

Providing patients with information has been high on the political and nursing agendas for many years. Over a decade ago the government addressed the issue with the *Patient's Charter* (DoH, 1991) by stating that hospitals should offer clear and sensitive explanations of clinical matters to patients. Subsequent documents have continued with the same aim, for example the *Patient Partnership Strategy* launched in 1996 by the NHS executive to enable patients to become informed about their treatment and care and the revised document published in 1999 *Patient and Public Involvement in the New NHS* (DoH, 1999b). These documents have continued to stress not only the importance of providing patient information but also getting patients involved in the production of that information.

Studies have shown that information can decrease postoperative pain, decrease the amount of opioid analgesia required, decrease anxiety and increase patient satisfaction (Egbert *et al.*, 1964; Hayward, 1975). More recently the analgesic reduction component of the earlier study findings has been disputed, although Callaghan *et al.* (1998) did reiterate reports that patients who had been adequately psychologically prepared preoperatively experienced less anxiety, lower stress levels and higher levels of satisfaction.

Patients clearly benefit from preoperative psychological preparation yet patients continue to arrive at theatre unprepared and highly anxious (Garretson, 2004). Patient ignorance and fear of what to expect with regard to postoperative pain and its control can increase both patient dissatisfaction and the degree of pain experienced in the postoperative period (Royal College of Anaesthetists (RCA), 2000). The RCA suggests that 100% of elective patients should receive information preoperatively about the planned method of pain and emetic control and 75% of emergency cases should receive the same service.

From a legal perspective practitioners are obliged to provide information that patients understand, not only about what a procedure involves but also how it may affect them in the future. Although verbal communication is essential to patient care it may not be sufficient on its own and literature should also be used. Useful patient guides relating to epidural analgesia have been produced by the RCA and are available on the RCA website.

REFERENCES

Callaghan, P., Yuk-Lung, C., King-Yu, Y. and Siu-Ling, C. (1998) The effect of preoperative information on post operative anxiety, satisfaction with information, and demand for analgesia in Chinese men having trans-urethral resection of the prostate (TURP). *Journal of Clinical Nursing,* **7** (5), 479–80.

Department of Health (1991) *The Patient's Charter.* London: Stationery Office.

Department of Health (1999a) *Clinical Governance: Quality in the NHS.* London: Stationery Office.

Department of Health (1999b) *Patient and Public Involvement in the New NHS.* London: Stationery Office.

Egbert, L., Battit, G., Welch, C. and Bartlett, M. (1964) Reduction of postoperative pain by encouragement and instruction of patients. A study of doctor patient rapport. *New England Journal of Medicine,* **270**, 825–7.

Fordham, A. (2005) Using a competency based approach in nurse education. *Nursing Standard,* **19** (31), 41–8.

Garretson, S. (2004) Benefits of preoperative information programmes. *Nursing Standard,* **18** (47), 33–7.

Hayward, J. (1975) *Information: A Prescription Against Pain.* London: RCN.

McMullan, M., Endacott, R., Gray, M. *et al.* (2003) Portfolios and assessment of competence, a review of the literature. *Journal of Advanced Nursing,* **41** (3), 283–94.

National Health Service (2004) *The NHS Knowledge and Skills Framework (NHS KSF) and the Development of Review Process.* Cardiff: Welsh Assembly Government.

Nursing and Midwifery Council (2002) *Code of Professional Conduct.* London: NMC.

Redman, R., Lenburg, C. and Hinton-Walker, P. (1999) Competency assessment, methods for implementation in nursing education. *Journal of Issues in Nursing.* Available at: www.nursingworld.org/ojin/topic/tpc_3htm (accessed March 2005).

Royal College of Anaesthetists (2000) *Raising the Standard Audit Recipe Book.* London: RCA.

12

Clinical Governance and Clinical Audit

RACHEL SWINGLEHURST

Clinical Nurse Specialist in Pain Management, Withybush Hospital,
Pembrokeshire, South Wales

Clinical governance has had a major impact on health care; its role is to ensure that patients throughout the United Kingdom receive high quality clinical care. Clinical audit provides a means of measuring these standards of care.

This chapter will provide an overview of clinical governance in relation to epidural practice. This will include patient involvement; clinical risk management; clinical audit, effectiveness and standard setting; evidence based medicine and continuing professional development.

CLINICAL GOVERNANCE

In the United Kingdom, the government has introduced a system for monitoring the quality of the National Health Service (NHS), this has been called clinical governance. Clinical governance has been reinforced by the statutory duty for quality that has been placed on all NHS organisations by the Health Act (DoH, 1999b). It is a framework through which NHS organisations are accountable for continuously improving the quality of their services by safeguarding high standards of care (DoH, 1998). However, Phipps (2000) suggests that once past the executive level where clinical governance is now part of

Epidural Analgesia in Acute Pain Management. Edited by Carolyn Middleton.
© 2006 by John Wiley & Sons, Ltd.   ISBN 0-470-01964-6

mainstream responsibilities, it is less clear how involved nurses and other professionals are in clinical governance issues. It is only when healthcare practitioners begin to reflect on how it will impact on their own clinical practice that it becomes real to individuals.

Making a Difference (DoH, 1999a), the national nursing strategy, focuses on how nurses can enhance the quality of care. It stresses the need for the involvement of the nursing professions in taking clinical governance forward with more involvement in research and development. The Royal College of Nursing (2003) suggests that the term clinical governance is a paradigm for everything that helps to maintain and improve standards of patient care including epidural infusions.

Epidural analgesia is an accepted medical intervention for the management of postoperative pain. To be clinically effective there are four main features that are required to be addressed within the clinical governance arena. These are:

1. patient involvement;
2. clinical risk management;
3. continuing professional development;
4. clinical audit, standard setting and evidence based medicine.

PATIENT INVOLVEMENT

The Wanless Report (2002) recommends that a more effective partnership between health professionals and the public be facilitated by the development of improved health information to help people engage with their care in an informed way. The Welsh Assembly's *Putting Public and Patient Involvement into Practice* (PPI) (2003) highlighted the innovations in care initiatives, fundamentals of care, CHI reviews, National Service Framework, care pathways, the creation of the National Patient Safety Agency and clinical governance developments. All these initiatives are intended to contribute to a new urgency for PPI which is now a key strand within clinical governance.

A small study by Quinn (2003) considered the patient perspective with regard to infusion devices. Having such a device as part of a patient's care is an unusual experience for patients who may require considerable emotional reassurance while the device is in use. Unfortunately nurses sometimes underestimate the intensity of patients' fears concerning such devices, this clearly is an area that needs to be addressed. Information can relieve anxiety, therefore patients should have the following information about the device given prior to its commencement.

- Why the patient requires the device.
- How long the device will be in place.

- The drugs and dosage used.
- Likely problems that may occur.
- Details of the devices used.

The participants of the Quinn (2003) study stressed that they were often worried when they heard the infusion device alarm for the first time. The noise was not only annoying but could also cause panic among those patients who assumed that it indicated a crisis. Moreover, the fact that the alarms went off frequently raised a fundamental issue of patient safety because sometimes the alarms would be ignored. Good communication for the patient regarding infusion devices is essential and it is good practice for verbal information to be backed up with good quality written leaflets such as those provided by the Royal College of Anaesthetists (available on the RCA website).

CLINICAL RISK MANAGEMENT

The main purpose of the DoH (2001) directive, Building a Safer NHS for Patients: Implementing an Organisation with a Memory, is to improve patient safety by reducing risk or harm through error. It stipulates that all trusts must have a protocol in place for reporting adverse events that identifies errors and risks in patient care. Professional bodies such as the Nursing and Midwifery Council (NMC) also outline nurses' responsibility in identifying and minimising risks to patients. The *Code of Professional Conduct* (NMC, 2002) states that nurses must work with other members of the healthcare team to promote healthcare environments for patients that are conducive to safe, therapeutic and ethical practice.

Possible risks

There are some possible risks associated with utilising epidural infusions which are outlined below.

- No dedicated infusion device for epidural analgesia.
- Infusion device used for various drug infusions which may increase the risk of the wrong drug being administered.
- Drug calculation errors due to a variety of different concentrations used in a trust.
- Delivery systems not locked when opioids are utilised.
- Delays in the continuation of infusion when bag or syringe requires change.
- Giving sets not colour coded for easy recognition.
- Giving sets that do not include an antisiphon system.
- No standardised training requirements for nurses and doctors.

Possible Standards

To avoid the potential risks a multidisciplinary working party should agree and implement standards which aim to minimise the risks for patients receiving an epidural infusion. These standards may include the following.

- Equipment locally should be standardised.
- Prefilled bags or syringes would prevent drug errors and/or calculation.
- Storage of prefilled bags or syringes locked in a controlled drugs (CD) cupboard, reducing the risk of the wrong solution being used.
- Devices should be lockable.
- Device should be dedicated for epidurals only.
- Colour coded dedicated giving sets used only for epidurals.
- Giving set must have an antisiphon system.
- Nurses and doctors trained to competency standard of the trust.
- Clinical guidelines for health professionals.

To help promote national guidelines, which would help to reduce local variations in healthcare delivery, the National Institute for Clinical Excellence (NICE) was established in 1999 (now, 2005, known as the National Institute for Health and Clinical Excellence). Its main function is to evaluate available evidence and produce clinical guidelines based on clinical efficacy and cost effectiveness. Research in the form of randomised controlled trials is generally thought to be the most reliable form of evidence (although factors relating to validity and reliability must be considered). NICE has stated that its clinical guidelines are intended to inform, not dictate practice and the guidelines need to bc updated as new evidence emerges, technology improves or expertise is gained (NICE, 2002, 2003). Unfortunately, at the present time NICE has not produced any guidelines specifically relating to epidural practice.

National benchmarking would be a useful way of enhancing clinical governance within the speciality of epidural practice. The advantage of benchmarking is that it helps to establish best practice and it allows the comparison of one service against another. Most importantly it allows the sharing of evidence (published and unpublished) and encourages research or audit in areas where little evidential support currently exists.

This book, which has been developed as a shared experience by clinical nurse specialists working in South Wales in the area of acute pain, will hopefully act as a best practice resource guideline for health professionals.

CONTINUING PROFESSIONAL DEVELOPMENT

Training in all aspects of epidural care for nurses and doctors should be based on competencies, which should be developed locally. As there may be some variation in such competencies this book can provide a framework of information to guide production of teaching plans An example of an appropriate competency based framework for nursing staff in relation to epidural management is set out in Chapter 11.

A clinical governance framework ought to improve the quality of care for patients receiving epidural infusion for pain management by delivering a safe and effective service by competent staff. It should acknowledge good practice and identify areas for improvement and so enhance the quality of patient care for all patients.

CLINICAL AUDIT, STANDARD SETTING AND EVIDENCE BASED MEDICINE

The concept of clinical audit is not new within the NHS, however with the introduction of clinical governance, audit has received greater prominence and even a central role within clinical practice. Clinical audit enables the assessment and improvement of clinical care against identified standards of best practice. It can be described as a cycle within which there are a number of stages that follow a systematic process (Figure 12.1).

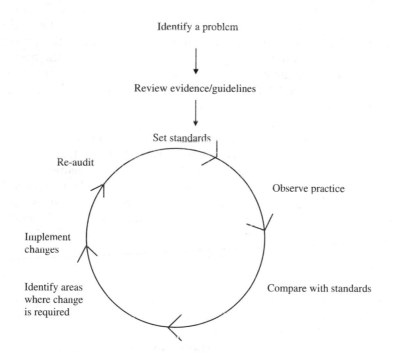

Figure 12.1. Evidence based clinical audit cycle. (From Clinical Audit Research Support Unit, Pembrokeshire and Derwen NHS Trust. Reproduced by permission of the Clinical Audit and Effectiveness Department at Withybush General Hospital.)

Before embarking on audit it is important to consider the differences between research and audit because they are sometimes confused. They utilise common approaches and analysis but the distinction is in their intention. The Royal College of Physicians (1996) suggests that in the most simplistic terms research is finding out about what ought to be done in clinical practice whereas audit is whether you are actually doing what you ought to be doing!

The best place to start an audit cycle is to establish good communication with other disciplines as audit is best carried out within a multidisciplinary perspective (Cooper and Benjamin, 2004). Next the focus of the audit must be determined along with identification of any relevant standards that are already available. National Framework documents, NICE guidelines and standards and guidelines published by professional bodies are some of the many sources available against which healthcare activities can be audited. However, there is a need not only to establish if such standards are evidence based but also to ensure that they are both definable and measurable.

Auditing acute pain management and epidural practice is problematic because of the lack of guidance and nationally agreed standards, therefore most in-patient pain services make local decisions about data to be collected. Where standards have been established against which an audit can be conducted, the next stage is to identify the data that are required. Once this has been done a data collection tool will need to be developed so the data can be collected. Following data collection it is important to consider the best way in which they should be analysed. The use of spreadsheets or even a database can be useful, often the Clinical Audit and Research Support Unit (CARSU) within a trust will help with the analysis.

Once analysis of the data has been performed the next step is to compare the findings against the identified standards and disseminate the results to the relevant individuals or departments involved. If the standards have not been met it will be necessary to identify areas where change is required, an action plan will need to be formed and plans for implementation drawn up. Often this is the most difficult stage in the audit process because people do not like change, however, involvement of the audit multidisciplinary team at every stage will hopefully motivate them to make the required changes in practice and therefore to have a stake in its success. Change needs to be sustained and re-audit undertaken in order to close the audit loop.

The Royal College of Anaesthetists (RCA) has produced a compendium of audit recipes for continuous quality improvement in anaesthesia, called *Raising the Standard*. These recipes have been developed as a tool to assist individuals and departments to undertake audit (RCA, 2000). Table 12.1 gives an example of an audit designed by the RCA and set out in its audit recipe book.

Table 12.1. Efficacy and safety on the postoperative ward audit. (From the Royal College of Anaesthetists (2002) *Raising the Standard*. Reproduced by permission of the Royal College of Anaesthetists)

Why do this audit?	Pain is a cause of postoperative morbidity and mortality. The *Report of the working party on pain after surgery* supports the use of analgesia systems such as patient controlled analgesia and epidurals in the general postoperative ward if supervised by an acute pain service (APS). Audit provides essential performance and safety feedback to guide the development of the service. The data are also useful when developing business plans to justify the service and its funding requirements
Best practice: research evidence or authoritative opinion	The poor provision of analgesia in 30–75% of surgical patients was well demonstrated and led to the widespread introduction of APS. The ward use of modern techniques of pain relief provides demonstrably better pain relief and may promote improved patient recovery
Suggested indicators	Existence of an APS in the hospital
	Percentage of postoperative patients who experience a failure of analgesia in the first 24 hours as defined below
	Percentage of patients in whom major and minor side effects occur
Proposed standard or target for best practice	There should be an APS in the hospital
	<1% postoperative patients should experience a failure of analgesia in the first 24 hours. In the absence of a nationally agreed pain scoring system, a score above 50% of the pain scale at two or more four hourly recordings in the first 24 hours constitutes a failure of analgesia. Pain should be assessed at rest and on movement (either coughing or touching the opposite side of the bed)
	The target for major and minor side effects should be in line with published data. These will vary according to the technique used. The following are examples for epidural opioids: pruritis, 30%; nausea, 30%; urinary retention, 15%; and respiratory depression, <1%

In conclusion, audit is a key part of clinical governance, the aim of which is to improve patient care by improving clinical practice. Clinical audit seeks to improve outcomes through the systematic review of care against explicit criteria and the implementation of change. To date, however, no national audits or guidelines exist in the United Kingdom regarding the management of acute pain and epidurals. Hopefully, in the future this will change with specialist nurses working within this field developing benchmarks to audit against, and so ensuring conformity of evidence based standards in epidural practice.

REFERENCES

Clinical Audit Research Support Unit, Pembrokeshire and Derwen NHS Trust Clinical audit cycle (Unpublished).

Cooper, J. and Benjamin, M. (2004) Clinical audit is practice. *Nursing Standard*, **18** (28), 47–53.

Department of Health (1998) *A First Class Service. Quality in the New NHS.* London: Stationery Office.

Department of Health (1999a) *Making a Difference (Nursing Strategy).* London: HMSO.

Department of Health (1999b) *Health Act.* London: Stationery Office.

Department of Health (2001) *Building a Safer NHS for Patients: Implementing an Organisation with a Memory.* London: Stationery Office.

National Institute for Health and Clinical Excellence (NICE) (2002) *Clinical Guidelines.* http://www.nice.org.uk (last accessed January 2005).

National Institute for Health and Clinical Excellence (NICE) (2003) *Fact Sheet: General Information About Clinical Guidelines.* London: NICE.

Nursing and Midwifery Council (2002) *Code of Professional Conduct.* London: NMC.

Phipps, K. (2000) Nursing and clinical governance viewpoint. *British Journal of Clinical Governance*, **5** (2), 69–70.

Quinn, C. (2003) Infusion devices: understanding the patient perspective to avoid errors. *Professional Nurse*, **19** (2), 79–83.

Royal College of Anaesthetists (2000) *Raising the Standard: a Compendium of Audit Recipes for Continuous Quality Improvement in Anaesthesia.* London: RCA.

Royal College of Nursing (2003) *Clinical Governance: an RCN Resource Guide.* London: RCN.

Royal College of Physicians of London (1996) *Guidelines on the Practice of Ethics Committees in Medical Research Involving Human Subjects*, 3rd edn. London: RCP.

Wanless, D. (2002) *The Wanless Report – Conclusions and Recommendations.* Available at: http://www.hm-treasury.gov.uk/media/C2BO6/chap7.pdf (last accessed 14/02/05).

Welsh Assembly Government (2003) *Putting Public and Patient Involvement into Practice.* Cardiff: Welsh Assembly.

Glossary

The following definitions are drawn from the chapters in this book and are intended as a resource for understanding.

Accountability – responsibility for one's actions.

Activated partial thromboplastin time – method of estimating the degree of anticoagulation induced by heparin therapy for venous thrombosis.

Acute pain management – the treatment of pain associated with tissue damage.

Adverse drug reactions – unexpected or unwanted side effects of a drug.

Adverse events – unwanted or unexpected event.

Ambulation – walking.

Anaesthetist – medically qualified doctor who administers anaesthetic to patient to induce unconsciousness before a surgical operation.

Analgesia – drug that relieves pain.

Analgesia – adjuvant – substance used in conjunction with another to enhance its activity.

Analgesia balanced – co-prescribing of analgesia as per the World Health Organisation Analgesic Ladder.

Analgesia failure – analgesia administered that does not relieve pain.

Analgesia inadequate – analgesia that only partially relieves pain.

Analgesia multi-modal approach – combination analgesics given in conjunction with each other to enhance analgesic effect.

Analgesia – pre-emptive – given prior to procedure.

Analgesia – regional – given directly to a specific anatomical area of the body.

Analgesia step down – graded reduction in analgesia in line with the World Health Organisation Analgesic Ladder.

Analgesic ladder – framework produced by the World Health Organisation for rational prescribing of pain killing drugs.

Epidural Analgesia in Acute Pain Management. Edited by Carolyn Middleton.
© 2006 by John Wiley & Sons, Ltd.   ISBN 0-470-01964-6

Anti-bacterial filter – device fitted into the epidural line that is designed to minimise the risk of intra-laminar bacterial contamination by excluding microscopic debris from epidural catheter.

Antibiotic – substance that destroys or inhibits the growth of a micro-organism.

Anticoagulant – agent that prevents the clotting of blood.

Anti-emetic – agent that prevents emesis (vomiting).

Anti-histamine drugs – agent that inhibits the action of histamine in the body by blocking histamine receptors.

Anti-siphon valve – device that prevents inadvertent siphoning of solution.

Aorto-caval compression/occlusion – condition that occurs in late stage of pregnancy where the uterus compresses the vena cava and aorta against the lumbar spine causing a reduction in venous return to the heart and a reduction in uterine blood flow.

Audit – process by which a systematic review of practice is examined.

Audit cycle – allows assessment and reassessment and improvement of clinical practice.

Audit data collection tool – document used to collect specific audit data.

Back pain – unpleasant sensation associated with actual or potential tissue damage arising from the spinal area.

Balanced analgesia – co-prescribing of pain killing drugs in line with the World Health Organisation Analgesic Ladder.

Benchmarking – a standard by which something can be measured.

Block – interruption of physiological function brought about intentionally as part of a therapeutic procedure.

Block – high block – block affecting dermatomes above intended level.

Block level – referring to the dermatomal levels affected by local anaesthetic.

Block testing – examining the extent of dermatomal spread of local anaesthetic.

Blood patch – technique involving epidural injection of autologous blood in an attempt to close a dural puncture.

Blood pressure – force exerted by the circulating blood against the walls of the arteries, veins and chambers of the heart.

Bolus administration – direct administration of pharmacological preparations.

Bolus dose size – measured amount of pharmacological preparation.

Bromage score – tool for measuring motor function of lower limbs in relation to administration of epidural analgesia.

Caesarean section – surgical operation for delivering a baby through the abdominal wall.

Cardio-respiratory arrest – ceasing of cardiac and respiratory functioning.

Cardio-respiratory resuscitation – an emergency procedure for life support consisting of artificial respiration and manual external cardiac massage.

Cardiovascular system – comprises the heart and circulatory system.

Catheter insertion – placing of the epidural catheter into the epidural space.

Catheter migration – inadvertent movement of the epidural catheter out of the epidural space into surrounding tissue.

Catheter removal – taking out of the body of an epidural catheter.

Central nervous system – consists of the brain and spinal cord.

Central nervous system toxicity – degree to which the central nervous system is poisoned by a substance.

Cephalad migration – inadvertent movement of the epidural catheter towards the head.

Cerebrospinal fluid – clear watery fluid that surrounds the brain and spinal cord contained in the sub arachnoid space.

Cerebrospinal fluid leakage – inadvertent escape of cerebrospinal fluid from the sub arachnoid space.

Chemo-receptor trigger zone – group of cells that responds to specific chemical compounds by initiating an impulse in a sensory nerve.

Clinical governance – a framework through which NHS organisations are accountable for continually improving the quality of their services and safeguarding high standards of care.

Clinical incident reporting – recording and reporting of adverse events.

Clinical management plan – framework used for supplementary prescribing.

Clinical nurse specialist – a nurse or midwife specialist in clinical practice (who) has undertaken formal recognised post-registration education relevant to his/her area of specialist practice.

Clinical risk management – method of minimising clinical risk.

Coagulation – the process by which a colloid liquid changes to a jelly-like mass.

Coagulopathy – a disease that affects the coagulability of blood.

Communication – impart, transmit or receive information.

Compartment syndrome – a condition that results from swelling within a compartment of a limb that raises the pressure so that blood supply to the muscle is cut off.

Competence – ability to do a task properly.

Competency based assessment – assessment of the performance of an individual measured against clearly defined outcomes.

Complications – condition arising during the course of or as a consequence of a process.

Confidentiality – information that will not be disclosed.

Conscious level – level of awareness of one's surroundings.

Consent – to agree to do something or allow another to carry out a procedure.

Continuing professional development – ongoing work related education.

Controlled drugs – medication controlled by the laws relating to drugs.

Controlled drugs register – book for recording usage of controlled medication.

Convulsions – to shake violently with sudden uncontrolled movements.

Co-prescribing – the prescribing of adjuvant therapy.

Dedicated lines – giving set specifically for administration of epidural infusions.

Deep vein thrombosis – obstruction of a deep vein by a blood clot.

Dermatomes – segmented areas of skin and deeper tissues innervated by spinal nerves.

Documentation – text that is written or stored/printed information.

Dosing regimen – medication administration recipe.

Drug error – inadvertent administration of the wrong drug or dose.

Drug toxicity – degree to which a substance is poisonous.

Dura breach – a hole in the dura mater.

Dura mater – thickest and outermost of the three meninges surrounding the brain and spinal cord.

Dura puncture – inadvertent hole made in the dura mater.

Education – systematic instruction or training.

Electro-biomedical engineering – engineering department that provides technical support and advice for epidural infusion devices or pumps.

Endogenous opioids – naturally occurring painkillers derived from the body.

Endorphins – one of a group of chemical compounds similar to encephalins that occur naturally in the brain and have pain-relieving properties.

Epidural abscess – localised collection of pus in the epidural space.

Epidural catheter – tube used to administer epidural solution into the epidural space.

Epidural catheter dislodgement – inadvertent movement of the epidural catheter from the epidural space.

Epidural catheter disconnection – inadvertent undoing of connection of the epidural catheter.

Epidural catheter falling out – inadvertent total removal of the epidural catheter from the epidural space.

Epidural catheter insertion – introduction of the epidural catheter into the epidural space.

Epidural catheter labelling – adhesive paper attached to the epidural catheter indicating its nature.

Epidural catheter leakage – leaking of epidural solution around the epidural catheter.

Epidural catheter migration – inadvertent movement of the epidural catheter out of the epidural space.

Epidural catheter multi fenestration – numerous holes that allow epidural solution to exit the epidural catheter.

Epidural catheter obstruction – blockage of the epidural catheter.

Epidural catheter occlusion – obstruction of the epidural catheter.

Epidural catheter removal – to take the epidural catheter out of the epidural space.

Epidural catheter technical problems – problems associated with the epidural delivery equipment.

Epidural catheter terminal eye – catheter with a single hole at the tip end of the catheter that allows epidural solution to exit the catheter into the epidural space.

Epidural catheter tip – the terminal end of the epidural catheter.

Epidural catheter tip inspection – the checking of the presence of the epidural catheter tip after removal of the catheter.

Epidural catheter tip sheared off – inadvertent breaking off of the end of the epidural catheter within epidural space.

Epidural catheter withdrawal – retraction of the epidural catheter by a specified length measurement.

Epidural caudal spread – movement of epidural solution into lower part of the epidural space.

Epidural cocktail – combination of drugs administered via the epidural catheter.

Epidural concentration – strength of the epidural solution.

Epidural contraindications for use – reasons for not using an epidural infusion.

Epidural cranial spread – movement of epidural solution toward the brain.

Epidural delivery systems – method of administering epidural solution.

Epidural device – pump used for the delivery of epidural solution.

Epidural indications for use – reasons for administering epidural solution.

Epidural space – anatomical area located between the dura mater and the vertebral canal.

Epidural vein insertion – inadvertent insertion of the epidural catheter into the epidural vein.

ESSAM block scoring tool – tool for assessing motor blockade of the upper limbs.

Evidence based medicine – care based on the best evidence from well constructed randomised controlled trials.

Exogenous source – originating from a source external to the body.

Fixative device – mechanism designed to perform specific function of holding epidural catheter in position.

Fluid balance – the difference between the amount of fluid taken into the body and the amount of fluid excreted or lost.

General anaesthetic – agent that reduces or abolishes sensation and consciousness of the whole body.

Gravitational effects – sinking movement of epidural cocktail by the force of gravity within the epidural space.

Guidance documents/guidelines – written instructions that provide principles and standards for epidural practice.

Haematoma – an accumulation of blood within the tissues that clots to form a solid swelling.

Hallucinations – false perceptions of something that is not really there.

Headache – pain felt deep within skull.

Hypotension – abnormally low arterial blood pressure.

Hypoventilation – breathing at an abnormally shallow or slow rate.

Hypovolaemia – decrease in volume of circulating blood.

Hypoxia – deficiency of oxygen in tissues.

Immuno-compromised – when the immune response is reduced or defective.

Infection – invasion of the body by a harmful organism.

Infection – **systemic** – infection affecting the whole body.

Information technology – the science and activity of using computers and other electronic equipment to store and send information.

Informed consent – consent by a patient to a procedure after achieving an understanding of the relevant medical facts and risks involved.

Infusion – **background** – continuous infusion of drug via a delivery device administered without requiring patient request.

Infusion – **bolus** – intermittent measured amount of administered drug.

Infusion – **complications** – problems associated with an epidural infusion.

Infusion – **continuous** – constant administration of drugs via a delivery device.

Infusion – **delivery mode** – method of administration of pharmacological infusion.

Infusion – **demand dose mode** – method of administration of pharmacological infusion that involves a patient request system.

Infusion device – pump used for the administration of pharmacological solutions.

Infusion – **duration** – length of time that an infusion will be in progress.

Infusion – **intermittent** – administration of an infusion on a periodic basis.

Infusion – **maximum** – highest set rate of drug administration.

Infusion – **patient controlled epidural analgesia** – administration that requires a patient operated demand button system.

Infusion – **rate** – measured amount of pharmacological infusion delivered in a set period of time.

Instrumental delivery incidence – vaginal delivery of a baby that requires instrumental assistance.

Intra-luminar bacterial contamination – contamination from within the epidural catheter.

Intra-thecal space – within the meninges of the spinal cord.

Intra-thecal catheter migration – inadvertent movement of the epdiural catheter through the dura into the intra-thecal space.

Knowledge and skills framework – a development tool to provide the basis of progression within agenda for change pay bands.

Labour – the sequence of events by which a baby and the afterbirth are expelled from the uterus at childbirth.

Legislation – legal directives.

Link nurse – ward based nurse who has close links with a specialist service i.e. the acute pain service.

Local anaesthetic adverse effects – unwanted or unexpected effects of local anaesthetic drugs.

Local anaesthetic/opioid combination – combination of both local anaesthetic and an opioid in an epidural mixture.

Local anaesthetic pharmaco-dynamics – the interaction of local anaesthetic with the body's cells.

Local anaesthetic pharmaco-kinetics – the study of how local anaesthetics are handled within the body.

Local anaesthetic toxicity – the degree to which a local anaesthetic is poisonous.

Lock box – security box used to store the epidural solution whilst the infusion is in progress.

Loss of resistance – technique used for identifying the epidural space.

Mobile epidural – epidural infusion that does not interfere with motor function and therefore allows mobilisation.

Monitoring – to watch and check a patient carefully in order to observe effects.

Motor blockade – effects of local anaesthetic on motor nerve fibres.

Multidisciplinary working – different healthcare disciplines working together.

Muscle weakness – lack of muscle power.

Naloxone – drug used for reversing the effects of respiratory depression.

Nausea – the feeling of being about to vomit.

Nerve cell – one of the basic functional units of the nervous system.

Nervous system – a vast network of cells which specialised in carrying information in the form of nerve impulses to and from all parts of the body.

Neurological deficit – a lacking of function of the nervous system.

Neuronal membrane – nerve cell membrane.

Neuropathy – disease of the peripheral nerves usually causing weakness and numbness.

Neuropathy – transient – short term weakness and numbness of the peripheral nerves.

Neurotransmitter – a chemical substance released from nerve endings to transmit impulses actors synapses to other structures including nerves.

Nociception – the conduction of pain.

Nociceptive fibres – nerve fibres which are responsible for the conduction of pain.

Non-pharmacological adjuncts – additional treatments that are not drug based.

Non steroidal anti-inflammatory drugs – a large group of drugs used for pain relief which have anti inflammatory properties.

Opioid – one of the group of drugs derived from opium.

Opioid antagonist – a drug that binds with opioid receptors but does not activate them.

Opioid pharmaco-dynamics – the interaction of opioids with the body's cells.

Opioid pharmaco-kinetics – the study of how opioids are handled within the body.

Opioid receptors – cell or group of cells that specialise in the detection of opioids.

Oral medication – drugs taken by mouth.

Oxygen – an odourless, colourless gas that makes up one fifth of the atmosphere and is essential to most life forms.

Paediatric – referring to children.

Pain – an unpleasant sensation that occurs in relation to tissue damage.

Pain assessment – method of establishing the intensity and location of pain.

Pain assessment CRIES – tool for assessing the intensity of pain in babies.

Pain assessment FACES – tool for assessing the intensity of pain in children.

Pain assessment multi-dimensional tool – tool that assesses all aspects of pain.

Pain assessment numerical rating scale – tool that assesses intensity of pain using a numerical scoring system.

Pain assessment one-dimensional tools – tool that assesses only one aspect of pain, usually intensity.

Pain assessment TPPPS – tool for assessing the intensity of pain in toddlers.

Pain assessment verbal rating scale – tool that assesses intensity of pain using a series of verbal descriptors.

Pain assessment visual analogue scale – tool that assesses intensity of pain using a horizontal line as a continuum which the patient marks to represent the intensity of pain.

Paracetamol – simple analgesic drug.

Paraesthesia – altered sensation.

Paralysis – muscle weakness that varies in extent.

Paraplegia – paralysis of both legs.

Peri-operative – during surgery.

Peripheral nerve palsy – paralysis.

Pharmacist – person who prepares and dispenses drugs.

Physiology – the science of the function of living organisms and their component parts.

Policy – a set of ideas or a plan of what to do in particular situations that has been agreed officially by a group of people.

Post dural puncture headache – headache that occurs following puncture of the dura.

Pre-emptive analgesia – painkillers given prior to a procedure in a bid to reduce pain post procedure.

Pre-operative – prior to surgery.

Prescribing – written directions from a registered medical practitioner to a pharmacist for preparing and dispensing a drug.

Prescribing – supplementary – prescribing by an allied health professional working to a clinical management plan set up by a medical prescriber.

Prescriptions chart – document on which medications are prescribed and administration of medications recorded.

Pressure sores – an ulcerated area of skin caused by continuous pressure.

Protocols – document that outlines a system of rules relating to a specific situation or procedure.

Pruritus – itching.

Pulmonary embolism – obstruction of the pulmonary artery or one of its branches by a blood clot.

Pulse – series of pressure waves within an artery caused by contractions of the left ventricle and corresponding with the heart rate.

Pulse oximetry – measurement of the proportion of oxygenated haemoglobin in the blood.

Pyrexia – a rise in body temperature above the normal.

Radiculopathy – pain, numbness, weakness and reflex loss in the limbs.

Record keeping – recording of information.

Regional anaesthesia – administration of local anaesthetic to a specific body area.

Research – detailed study of a subject.

Respiratory depression – low respiratory rate (below 8 breaths per minute)

Respiratory rate – breathing rate, e.g. number of breaths taken per minute.

Resuscitation – the restoration of a breathing and cardiac function.

Risk – to do something although there is a chance of a bad result.

Sedation – production of a restful state of mind.

Sensory loss – reduction in incoming sensory information.

Sepsis – the destruction of tissues by disease causing bacteria or their toxins.

Skin preparation – appropriate cleansing and decontamination of the skin prior to epidural catheter insertion.

Spinal anatomy – components of the spinal column.

Spinal cord – portion of the central nervous system enclosed in the vertebral column consisting of nerve cells and bundles of nerves connecting all parts of the body with the brain.

Spinal cord compression – increased pressure on the spinal cord.

Spinal cord decompression – surgical reduction of pressure on the spinal cord.

Spinal nerve – nerve that leaves the spinal cord and is distributed to the body.

Spinal nerve root – part of the nerve that passes from the vertebral canal through the spaces between the arches of the vertebrae.

Standard setting – setting of criteria by which healthcare is measured.

Stress response – specific physiological actions in the sympathetic nervous system, primarily caused by release of adrenaline and norepinephrine from the medulla of the adrenal glands.

Sub-arachnoid space – space between the arachnoid and pia mater.

Sub-dural haematoma – accumulation of blood below the dura mater that clots to form a solid swelling.

Sub-dural space – space between the dura and arachnoid mater.

Supine hypotensive syndrome – combination of signs and symptoms relating to abnormally low arterial blood pressure when the patient is in a laying position.

Supplementary prescribing – prescribing by an allied health professional working to a clinical management plan.

Sympathetic blockade – application of local anaesthetic to the sympathetic nervous system.

Sympathetic nerve supply – fibres that leave the nervous system via a chain of ganglia close to the spinal cord in the thoracic and lumbar regions.

Sympathetic nervous system – one of the two divisions of the autonomic nervous system.

Synergistic effect – combined analgesic effects that is greater than the individual pharmacological components.

Systemic migration – inadvertent movement of epidural catheter into the circulatory system, e.g. via an epidural vein.

Temperature – degree of body heat.

Test dose – small dose of pharmacological preparation administered in order to assess efficacy and associated adverse drug reactions.

Thrombocytopaenia – reduction in the number of platelets in the blood.

Thrombo-prophylaxix – agent that prevents the development of blood clots.

Titration – to determine volumetric quantity required by adding agents of known strength until desired effect is reached.

Top-up bolus – administration of a set volume of pharmacological preparation.

Total spinal anaesthesia – high plasma concentrations of free local anaesthetic resulting in central nervous system toxicity.

Training – mandatory – authoritative command from a superior for specific education.

Training – statutory – education imposed by law.

Trouble shooting – to identify problems and their potential solutions.

Tunnelled catheters – epidural catheter that is burrowed subcutaneous away from the insertion site.

Tuohy needle – needle used to introduce the epidural catheter into the epidural space.

Uterine contractions pain – shortening of the uterine muscles in response to a motor nerve impose which generates tension in the uterine muscles.

Urinary catheterisation – introduction of a drainage tube into the bladder via the urethra.

Urinary incontinence – inappropriate involuntary passage of urine.

Urinary output – amount of urine voided.

Urinary retention – inability to pass urine that is retained in the bladder.

Vasoconstriction – decrease in diameter of blood vessels especially arteries.

Vasodilation – increase in the diameter of blood vessels especially arteries.

Vasopressors – drug that stimulates the contraction of blood vessel therefore bringing about an increase in blood pressure.

Venous air embolism – air that obstructs the outflow of blood from the right ventricle of the heart.

Vertebrae – bones that make up the spinal column.

Vomiting – the reflex action of ejecting the contents of the stomach through the mouth.

Index